NATURAL WEIGHT LOSS

The Prevention Total Health System®

NATURAL WEIGHT LOSS

by the Editors of
Prevention® Magazine

 Rodale Press, Emmaus, Pennsylvania

Copyright © 1985 by Rodale Press, Inc.

All rights reserved. No part of this publication may be reproduced or transmitted in any form or by any means, electronic or mechanical, including photocopy, recording, or any information storage and retrieval system, without the written permission of the publisher.

Printed in the United States of America on recycled paper containing a high percentage of de-inked fiber.

Library of Congress Cataloging in Publication Data

Main entry under title:

Natural weight loss.

(The Prevention total health system)
Includes index.
1. Reducing diets. 2. Health.
I. Prevention (Emmaus, Pa.) II. Series.
RM222.2.N375 1985   613.2′5   84-15993
ISBN 0-87857-529-4 hardcover
    6 8 10 9 7 5   hardcover

NOTICE

This book is intended as a reference volume only, not as a medical manual or guide to self-treatment. If you suspect that you have a medical problem, we urge you to seek competent medical help. Keep in mind that nutritional and health needs vary from person to person, depending on age, sex, health status and total diet. The information here is intended to help you make informed decisions about your health, not as a substitute for any treatment that may have been prescribed by your doctor.

The Prevention Total Health System®

Series Editors: William Gottlieb, Mark Bricklin
Natural Weight Loss Editor: Debora Tkac
Writers: William Ehrhart (Chapter 1), Stephen Williams (Chapters 2, 5), Marian Wolbers (Chapters 3, 6), Susan DeMark (Chapters 4, 8), Sharon Faelten and Debora Tkac (Chapter 7), Nona Cleland (Chapter 9)
Research Chief: Carol Baldwin
Associate Research Chiefs, Prevention Health Books: Susan Nastasee, Christy Kohler
Researchers: Tawna Clelan, Holly Clemson, David Palmer, Carole Rapp, Sue Ann Alleger, Martha Capwell, Freda Christie, Jan Eickmeier, Amy Jordan
Food Consultants: Tom Ney, Director, Rodale Food Center; Anita Hirsch, Supervisor of Publication Testing; Linda C. Gilbert, Manager of Product Development
Copy Editor: Jane Sherman
Copy Coordinator: Joann Williams
Series Art Director: Jerry O'Brien
Art Production Manager: Jane C. Knutila
Designers: Lynn Foulk, Alison Lee
Illustrators: Bascove, Susan M. Blubaugh, Joe Lertola, Donna Ruff, Mary Anne Shea
Associate Designer: John Pepper
Project Assistant: Lisa Gatti
Director of Photography: T. L. Gettings
Photo Editor: Margaret Skrovanek
Photographic Stylists: Barbara Fritz, Renee R. Grimes, Kay Seng Lichthardt, Laura Hendry Reifsnyder, Scott Schmidt, J. C. Vera
Photo Researcher: Donna Lewis
Staff Photographers: Christopher Barone, Angelo M. Caggiano, Carl Doney, Mitchell T. Mandel, Alison Miksch, Margaret Skrovanek, Sally Shenk Ullman
Production Manager: Jacob V. Lichty
Production Coordinator: Barbara A. Herman
Composite Typesetter: Brenda J. Kline
Production Administrator: Eileen F. Bauder
Office Personnel: Susan K. Lagler, Diana M. Gottshall, Carol Petrakovich, Cindy Harig, Marge Kresley, Connie Shollenberger

Rodale Books, Inc.
Publisher: Richard M. Huttner
Senior Managing Editor: William H. Hylton
Copy Manager: Ann Snyder
Art Director: Karen A. Schell
Director of Marketing: Pat Corpora
Business Manager: Ellen J. Greene
Continuity Marketing Manager: John Taylor

Rodale Press, Inc.
Chairman of the Board: Robert Rodale
President: Robert Teufel
Executive Vice President: Marshall Ackerman
Group Vice Presidents: Sanford Beldon
                       Mark Bricklin
Senior Vice President: John Haberern
Vice Presidents: John Griffin
                 Richard M. Huttner
                 James C. McCullagh
                 David Widenmyer
Secretary: Anna Rodale

Contents

Planning for the New You

Every culture has health challenges that demand preventive action.

In some parts of the world, it's malnutrition. Or parasites. Or insanitary water supplies. They may not kill outright, but they sap vitality, undercut personal productivity and open the door to other health problems.

It's different, of course, in our own culture—but somehow the same. We, too, have an endemic condition that saps the energy and performance of millions, that sets us up for even bigger problems.

It's overweight.

Overweight—I hate the word *obesity*—is no sin. No more than anemia in an Indian farmer. It jumps at us from the everyday world we live in and those of us who are unlucky enough to be vulnerable—well, we get fat.

Overweight isn't caused by a germ, but in many ways it does come with the modern territory. Eve may have tripped up on the apple and had to start wearing a fig-leaf bikini in shame, but today's woman has to contend with apple pie that contains almost four times the calories. She'd be *glad* to slip into a fig-leaf bikini—if it would only fit!

Is apple pie *evil*? No. But it seems many of us are no better equipped to deal with the temptation of rich foods than we are with the temptation of sin. Neither are mice. Give the average rodent a diet of super-healthy mousie chow and he'll eat no more than he needs. But fill his feeding tray with a gorgeous buffet of human-style goodies, and he'll do the same thing we would. Blimp out. And get fat. Just like us.

I call it the Cornucopia Trap. For 99.9 percent of our time on earth, our big nutrition problem was getting enough to eat. Now, when so much artfully prepared food is available to all, the instincts that kept us energized and healthy through tough times are operating to do just the opposite.

This holdover from the "Wow, food!" syndrome is only half the story. The other half is "Ugh, work!" Everything from elevators and escalators to computers and remote-controlled TV. It all says the same thing: Stay put; I'll do it for you. So just when we have all the food—and *more*—we need to fuel our physical work, we don't have enough physical work to do.

Hello, diet.

Yes, hello, diet, and goodbye, peace of mind. Goodbye, health of body. Goodbye, joy of eating.

Goodbye, diet. Hello, Natural Weight Loss.

No, this book isn't a diet. Diets, I firmly believe, will go down in medical history along with other unnatural acts like enemas and tonsillectomies, as trendy ideas unmasked as mindless fads.

What we offer here is a systematic, holistic approach to weight control that is a natural part of the safe, sensible lifestyle approach that makes up The Prevention Total Health System.® It's the system I used some years ago to lose 30 pounds, and it has kept the new clothes I bought then from being confined to the Museum of Nice Tries.

Whether you want to lose weight, as I did, or maintain your current weight, this volume of our Prevention Total Health System® should open new vistas of self-improvement to you. It's a new approach to a New You.

Executive Editor, **Prevention**® Magazine

1

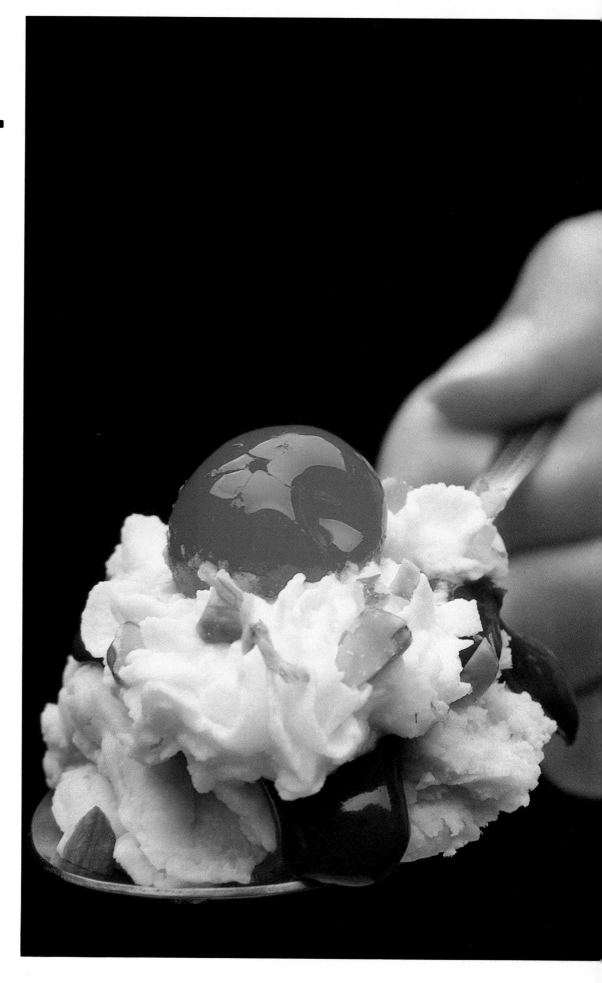

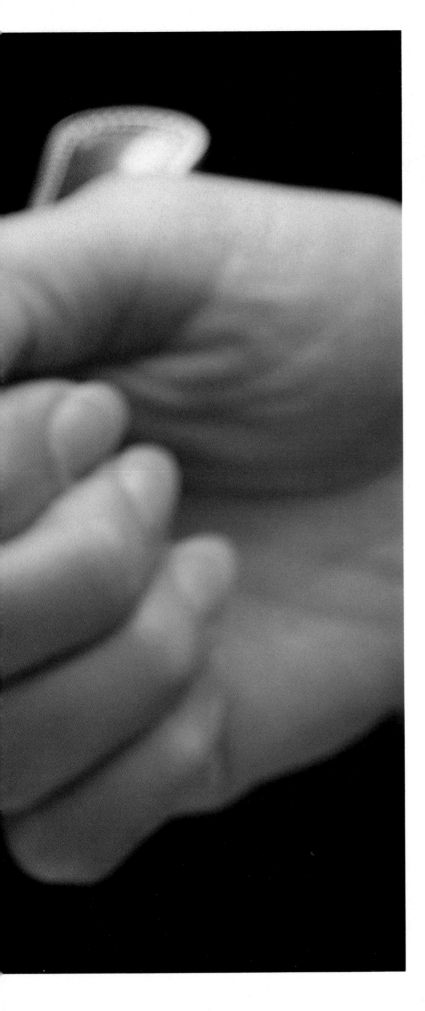

Overweight: A Lifestyle Out of Balance

History shows that as modern technology geared up, our bodies slowed down—and spread out. It's a problem you can overcome.

Forty years ago, in the wintry Ardennes forest of western Europe, American soldiers and their Allied compatriots fought a great struggle that came to be known as the Battle of the Bulge. The fighting was desperate, and for a few days the outcome was in doubt. But eventually the tide was turned, the Allies were victorious, and they swept on to ultimate victory in World War II.

Today, Americans are engaged in another "battle of the bulge." While it is far less dramatic and its outcome can't be determined in the course of a few days, or even a few weeks or months, evidence of the struggle is everywhere. You can see it in the proliferation of health spas, racquetball clubs and sidewalk joggers; in bookstores featuring a succession of diet books and exercise books sizzling on the bestseller list; in fast food restaurants that now include salad bars; and in supermarkets bursting with low-calorie this and low-fat that.

Make no mistake about it: This is no mere tempest in a teapot, for Americans as a group are indeed bulging. A National Health and Nutrition Examination Survey conducted a few years ago determined that 32 percent of adult men and 36 percent of adult women were 10 percent or more above average weight. Nor has the situation improved; indications are that the incidence of overweight is still rising. By any standard of measure, obesity is commonplace in the United States.

Reliable statistics on the prevalence of obesity in the United States only go back 30 or 40 years. But there is good evidence that shows creeping weight gain has been following Americans for more than a century. Statistics show that an average military service recruit in his early thirties who entered the Union Army in 1863 weighed about 147 pounds for his 5' 10'' height. By 1972, the U.S. male of similar age, with an average height of 5' 10'', was up to 176 pounds—a gain of 29 pounds. Why? Increased American reliance on machine labor is one reason.

The American diet—which now contains more fat and sugar and less complex carbohydrates and fiber than yesteryear—is another. But there is a glimmer of light in all this. Recent statistics show that the average weight of this male age group has dropped 3 pounds. Perhaps the fitness revolution and a new awareness of what we eat has something to do with it.

Most of us who *are* overweight, however, don't need anyone to tell us about it. All we need to do is look in the mirror. What people want to know is, what can be done about it? In short, can we win the battle of the bulge?

The answer is simple—yes. "Most people *can* lose weight or prevent weight gain," insists Bernard Gutin, Ph.D., professor of applied physiology and education at Columbia University's Teachers College. That's what this book is all about. It's not a diet book and it's not an exercise book, though it will tell you about diet and exercise. It's a book about weight loss—how to lose weight and, more important, how to *keep* it off.

But before we can begin to get rid of fat, it's important to know what it is and where it comes from. Only by understanding the causes of the problem can we begin to solve it.

FAT AND SURVIVAL

Do you ever get angry with your body for behaving the way it does? Almost as if it had "a mind of its own"? Well, in a way, it does. And you shouldn't get angry with it; it's only doing what it's been programmed to do over millions of years of evolution. We probably wouldn't even *be* here now if human beings didn't get fat! Let's take a closer look.

All mammals are very suscepti-ble to temperature fluctuations. We function optimally only within a very narrow range of temperatures, and even minor changes in body temperature can have profound effects on health and survival. To protect against this, most mammals insulate themselves with fur. But human beings have developed a different system. Instead of fur, we have a layer of fat just beneath the skin that regulates and controls our body temperature.

It's a very efficient system. Not only does it provide good insulation, but it has other advantages as well. Our body's fat supply serves as a kind of food bank, containing up to 90 percent of the body's energy reserves. When food is plentiful, the body stores extra energy in the form of fat; when food is scarce, the body converts this fat into fuel for heat and energy.

It's this system that has helped us survive. For most of human existence, we lived by hunting and gathering—much as the !Khung Bushmen of southern Africa's Kalahari Desert do today. Periodic times of plenty were interspersed among long periods of hunger.

"Someone would kill an antelope or a deer," explains Arnold Fox, M.D., author of *The Beverly Hills Medical Diet,* "and everybody would eat. Then there wouldn't be any food for a long time." Thus, the ability to store and burn fat was absolutely essential. Even after most humans gave up their nomadic ways and became farmers, beginning about

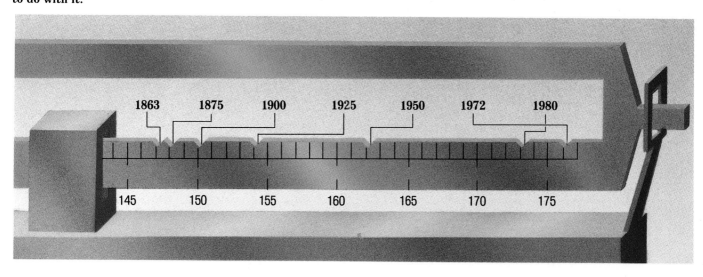

1863 1875 1900 1925 1950 1972 1980

145 150 155 160 165 170 175

Living Off the Fat of the Land

If the adult population of this country clambered up on a scale together, we'd weigh in at 2.3 billion pounds overweight. We're so overweight, in fact, that if we took the energy required to supply the food that keeps us fat and turned it into electricity, we could light up all the houses in Boston, Chicago, San Francisco and Washington, D.C., for a year!

Who's making light of the fat? Two scientists at the University of Illinois, Bruce M. Hannon, Ph.D., and Timothy G. Lohman, Ph.D. They calculated that we should shed 5.5 trillion excess calories in a national orgy of undereating. This would lead to energy savings equivalent to 1.3 billion gallons of gasoline. Once we were all semiactive

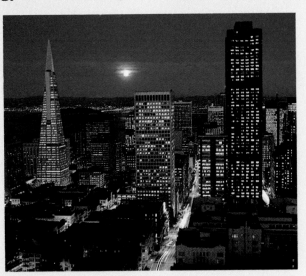

and of normal weight, we could eat at a maintenance level that would save about 3.5 trillion calories a year. In energy terms, that would free up enough gas to feed the tanks of 900,000 cars every year.

Dr. Hannon and Dr. Lohman are hoping that their findings provide the energy to switch on a light bulb in our national consciousness. When they look at a forkful of food, they don't see just chicken salad. Instead, they see the expenditure of energy that went into raising, feeding, processing, transporting, selling, buying and cooking the chicken. They'd like the rest of us to think of overeating in that way, too, and begin to conserve our national resources at the point where fork meets lip.

10,000 years ago, food supplies remained precarious and undependable, and times of want and famine were regular occurrences.

But technology changed all that—at least among Western cultures. Especially in the last century, modern agricultural techniques have made food both plentiful and relatively inexpensive. In the United States, the process has accelerated to the point where tempting, tasty food is readily available from vending machines, the household refrigerator, neighborhood supermarkets and fast food restaurants—that is to say, virtually anywhere and everywhere we turn.

The consequences are enormous, both figuratively and literally. "Human beings are built to be very efficient

at storing fat," explains David A. Levitsky, Ph.D., of Cornell University's department of psychology. "Until relatively recently, we never had to worry about *excess* food." One can imagine how a Bushman would react to a modern supermarket—or even the average home refrigerator. But we don't have to imagine it. Dr. Levitsky cites studies done with aboriginal Australians, Alaskan Eskimos and South American Indians. When hunter-gatherer people who are used to a subsistence life suddenly are incorporated into modern societies where food is plentiful, he says, they rapidly become obese. Some primordial mechanism buried deep within the body seems to say, "Hey, food! Better store all the fat I can *now*

(continued on page 6)

Body Images through the Ages

There are short, pudgy women, long, thin women and some women whose bodies don't leave any impression at all. Without a doubt, bodies come in numerous shapes and sizes—some determined by our hereditary genes, but all judged by our blue jeans. While it's in to be thin today, that wasn't necessarily the ideal of the yesterdays and may not be for the tomorrows. Over the decades—in fact, throughout the ages—the image of the ideal female body has gone through remarkable transition.

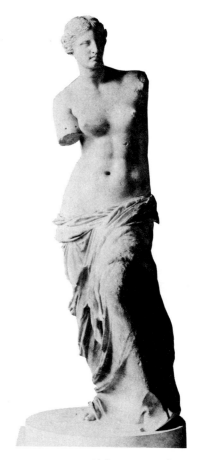

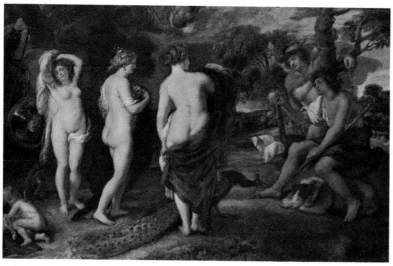

For a lot of women, life would be easier if the likes of Peter Paul Rubens were around today. The perfect body in the eyes of Rubens and others in the Baroque era of the late 1500s and early 1600s would never make it to the cover of today's magazines—unless it happened to be a publication for "big, beautiful women." But the voluptuous woman was clearly *the* image of a former era, as can be attested by this famous painting, *The Judgment of Paris* (1638-39), which now hangs in Madrid's Prado Museum.

Arms or no arms—this woman just wouldn't make it as today's ideal. But Venus de Milo, the ancient statue of Aphrodite, was obviously the epitome of womanhood when she was carved by an unknown sculptor of Antioch around 150 B.C. and even later in the 1800s when she was found on the island of Melos. For she became known as Venus, a name associated with charm, winsomeness and beauty. Nevertheless, today she can still turn a head in Paris's Louvre.

No wonder Scarlett O'Hara was such an obstinate woman. Anyone who had to have a trio of slaves tug on her corset laces to whittle her down to a 16-inch waist had a right to throw a tantrum or two! But that was the way of Civil War days, when having anything bigger than an 18-inch waist was just more than a young maiden could bear.

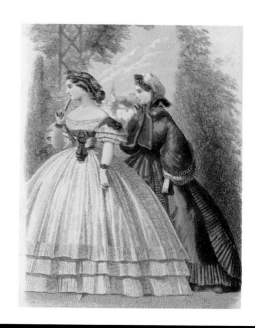

Boyish femininity—this was the quality that typified the ideal woman of the 1920s flapper era. After World War I when women won the right to vote, the young females of the time displayed their bold freedom of conviction through their conduct and dress—mannish bobs and loose-waisted dresses were the style of the day. To deemphasize their womanly curves, they bound their chests with strips of cloth, and some even used girdles to achieve the flat-chested, straight-bodied look you see here.

Today you might recognize this person as the woman who plugs the "full-figured look" (pity the poor ladies!) in lingerie commercials. But back in the 1940s when Jane Russell catapulted to fame, full-figured was *the* look *every* woman wanted to have. In fact, Howard Hughes, who produced the movie *The Outlaws,* which made her famous, designed a special bra—the cantilevered bra—to accentuate what was considered her finest quality. If such a body in such a bathing suit were to pose on a diving board today, the only reaction she would be liable to get from the photographer might be, "Please jump in."

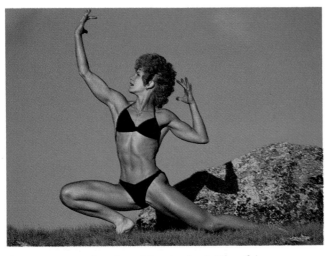

Any woman who dared try to look like this a generation or two ago would have people talking about her behind her back! Women were about as alien to sweat and gyms then as they are to corsets and bustles today. But weight lifting and body building are no longer male domains. In fact, the fit and flabless female body is considered downright sexy. Anyone for a workout?

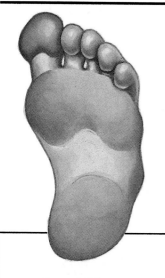

Be Kind to Your Feet

When a podiatrist suggests you take a load off your feet, he may not want you to sit down. He may want you to *slim* down.

Excess weight and foot problems go together. When feet are called on to carry a heavy burden of weight, those calluses and bunions will start radiating their discomfort. The delicate bone structure of the feet may realign under the added pressure, and knee pain can result. So can leg cramps, low back pain, corns, heel spurs, bursitis and arthritis.

The road from footloose to footsore is paved with excess weight.

because there's no telling when this gravy train will come to a screeching halt."

Okay, you say, but I'm not a hunter-gatherer suddenly turned loose in the local convenience store. True—but that primitive person is *inside* of you, programmed into your genes by evolution. And he's a lot more insistent than the conscious mind that tells you *not* to have that cheesecake. As Jean Himms-Hagen, Ph.D., of the department of biochemistry at the University of Ottawa, points out, "There's a great deal more obesity in affluent societies, and this surely has to do with the availability of food." The populations of many developing countries are much leaner than comparable groups in the United States.

DENSE CALORIES

But we don't have to look back to the dawn of history to see the problems that "progress" has brought. We need only compare our diet today with that of our ancestors just 80 years ago. The contemporary American diet includes a lot more sugar and fat, a lot fewer complex carbohydrates like whole grains and beans and far less dietary fiber. This increase in sugar, fat and simple carbohydrates has led to a more calorically dense diet—that is, you get more calories per volume of food eaten. It's easy to eat too much on a calorically dense diet because by the time your stomach fills up and says, "Stop, please, I'm stuffed; don't make me eat any more," you've already eaten far more than you need.

In contrast, fiber-rich diets like those earlier generations ate are more calorically dilute; you can get more bulk with fewer calories. Your stomach fills up before you've given yourself a caloric overdose. (Write down the number of times you've stuffed yourself silly on raw carrots or cauliflower in the past year. Now do the same thing with potato chips. Which figure is larger?) Foods high in fiber also generally require more chewing; this may cause you to eat more slowly, which helps prevent overeating.

How we eat matters, too. "We're a hurry-up society," says Dr. Fox. "It takes at least 20 minutes for the stomach to tell the brain that it's had enough to eat. But who takes 20 minutes for a meal these days? It's easier to open a can or put prepared food in the oven. A lot of people eat out two or even three meals a day, and they don't choose very carefully." A couple of cheeseburgers, french fries and a soda on the run represent a lot of calories in all the wrong forms.

Alcohol doesn't help, either. On the average, about 10 percent of our caloric intake comes from alcohol—and that 10 percent represents pure calories with virtually no nutritional value whatsoever.

And food and drink intake is only half the equation. While food has become increasingly available and the kinds of food we eat have been changing, our need to exert ourselves—to burn up the food we eat in the form of energy and heat—has steadily declined. We no longer chop wood, plow fields behind a team of oxen or grind our own flour by hand. We wear down-filled jackets and live in houses heated with oil, gas or electricity and insulated with fiberglass.

The fact is, we have to go out of our way to exert ourselves these days. "We don't even walk anywhere," says Dr. Fox. "In California, you're lost without a car, and it's not much better elsewhere."

"We're a mechanized society," says Thomas Wadden, Ph.D., of the University of Pennsylvania's department of psychiatry. "I recently heard that every time you put an extension phone in your house, you save 70 miles of walking a year. Is that good? I don't think so."

"When I was a child in the Bronx, we didn't have elevators," remembers Dr. Gutin, coauthor of *The High Energy Factor.* "There was only one building in our neighborhood that had one. We used to call it 'the elevator building.'" Today, you can't avoid them. Most high-rise office buildings have fire-locks on the stairwells, and even two-story department stores have escalators to carry shoppers from one floor to the other. And that's not all, by a long shot. We have machines to do our laundry, telephones with push-button dialing, even mechanical toothbrushes.

While the impact of any one of these labor-saving devices may not be too great, the cumulative effects are enormous.

In the past 30 years, labor-saving devices have cut up to 800 calories a day from our energy needs. The automatic dishwasher, for example, can add an extra 2 pounds a year. Having two or more cars for your family can add 10 pounds a year. Even a secretary who switches from a manual to an electric typewriter without reducing daily food intake can put on more than 5 pounds in a single year.

So it appears that the headlong advance of civilization has overtaken the ponderous pace of evolution, and the very mechanisms that permitted us to survive over thousands and even millions of years have become a severe burden for modern citizens faced with the bounty and blessings of technology.

But if *all* of us have outstripped evolution, how is it that some of us look like hippos while others are as lean as greyhounds? Well, there's no single answer, as you'll find out in a moment. But almost all the possible explanations have one thing in common: *You* are in charge of your weight. You're not at the mercy of bloated genes, a preordained body type of the Santa Claus variety or a fat virus that infected you at birth. Your weight is controllable—by you.

There are exceptions, of course. Some obese people suffer from faulty endocrine systems, tumors of the hypothalamus or hereditary disorders, says Veronica K. Piziak, M.D., Ph.D., associate professor of endocrinology at Texas A & M University College of Medicine. But such disorders affect only 1 to 2 percent of obese people. What about the rest of us?

Well, there's no one cause that sticks out like a sore thumb. It's more like a hand with two or three sore fingers.

"Obesity is not a single disease," says Judith S. Stern, Sc.D., professor of nutrition and director of the food intake laboratory at the University of California at Davis, "For a given overweight individual, you have to look at the individual, the family, all sorts of factors." Adds Dr. Gutin, "If you try to isolate one factor to explain all cases of obesity, you miss the point. There are lots of factors."

IS OVERWEIGHT INHERITED?

One of those "sore fingers" is pointing accusingly at an overweight person's *parents*. According to Barbara E. Echols and Jay M. Arena, M.D., authors of *The Commonsense Guide to Good Eating*, children with two obese parents have an 80 percent chance of becoming obese, children with one obese parent have a 40 percent chance of becoming obese and children with both parents of normal weight have only a 10 percent chance of becoming obese.

Does this mean obesity is genetic—that you're stuck with two blue eyes and two love handles? "Fatness follows family line," concedes Stanley M. Garn, Ph.D., professor of human nutrition and anthropology at the University of Michigan, "and this would suggest a genetic model were it not true for *adopted* children also. But even adopted children tend to become obese if their adoptive parents are obese."

Dr. Garn suggests that fatness may be "learned behavior," that children pick up bad eating habits and patterns of inactivity from their parents. And learned behavior can be *un*learned. "Obese people even tend to have obese pets," he reports. "How do you explain that by genetics?!"

Aging appears to be another possible factor in weight gain. For many Americans, there is both a gradual accumulation of weight between the ages of 20 and 50 and an increase in fat as a percentage of body weight, despite the fact that people eat less as they age. But is this gain really an inevitable function of age? Not necessarily. Our level of activity appears to play a major role in weight control and aging. The "increase in body fat

Slimness: More Than Vanity

The payoff you'll get from keeping fit and trim goes far beyond what you'll ever see in the mirror. You can prevent some of the diseases and problems that have been linked to obesity, such as:
- Depression
- Diabetes mellitus
- Gallstones
- Congestive heart failure
- Hernias
- High blood pressure
- Kidney stones
- Menstrual disorders
- Osteoarthritis
- Stroke
- Certain types of cancer
- Toxemia of pregnancy
- Varicose veins, arteries or lymph vessels

with age is smaller in persons who continue to do heavy physical work throughout their lives," reports Theodore B. Van Itallie, M.D., of Columbia University's College of Physicians and Surgeons.

SETPOINT: A THERMOSTAT FOR BODY FAT

Another recent explanation for overweight is the setpoint theory. According to William Bennett, M.D., and Joe Gurin, authors of *The Dieter's Dilemma*, everyone has a control system that dictates how much fat to carry. The system, according to the theory, works like a thermostat for the body, and each person's setting is different. Your setpoint, say Dr. Bennett and Gurin, is "the weight you normally maintain, give or take a few pounds, when you're not thinking about it."

Because of your setpoint, when you try to lose weight by dieting, your body rebels. The mechanism starts working to make you feel hungry all the time, forcing you to eat more until you get back to the fat level dictated by your setpoint. It also slows down your metabolism, so you burn fewer calories. The reverse happens when you try to gain weight beyond your setpoint.

But Dr. Bennett and Gurin concede that one's setpoint isn't chiseled in stone. They suggest that you can move your setpoint up by eating rich, high-fat foods and sweets; conversely, they say exercise "seems to function as a handle to crank down the setting." Maybe they should call it a "sit-point" instead.

THE FIGURES DON'T LIE

So, why are some people fat and others lean? Actually, the answer is maddeningly simple, a matter of caloric mathematics. Whether we gain or lose weight, explains Dr. Stern, is "just a question of energy balance." Evolution, technology, setpoints and psychology aside, energy balance has been the governing force regulating body weight since the dawn of humanity.

It works like this: If you eat more than you need, the excess energy is stored as fat; if you eat less than you need, your body dips into its fat stores to make up the difference; if you eat exactly what you need, your weight remains stable. That's all there is to it.

"Well, if it's all so simple, wise guy," you're probably muttering right about now, "why can't I lose weight? I've tried every diet in every book, but nothing seems to work—not for long, at least."

Ah, but you haven't tried *this* book. And the fact is, there's little point in trying a "diet" at all. Are you ready for this? Going on a diet won't work! At least not if that's *all* you do. "Only 5 percent of patients who rely solely on diet can be expected to reach and maintain their optimal weight," says William E. Straw, M.D., of Palo Alto Medical Foundation and Stanford University Medical School. Weight-reduction programs fail 95 percent of the time.

Why? For one thing, says Dr. Gutin, "a diet is something you go on, and when you go off it the weight almost always returns because your lifestyle hasn't changed." For another thing, adds Dr. Straw, after a short while on a reduced-calorie diet, body forces tend to reduce basal metabolic rate—the energy you use when you're doing nothing at all except breathing, pumping blood and maintaining body temperature (all of which can account for as much as 60 percent of your total energy expenditure)—thereby reducing the effectiveness of the caloric deficit.

In other words, says Dr. Straw, the less you eat, the more your body slows down to compensate. This may be the setpoint mechanism in operation, or it may be the body's evolutionary response toward conservation of energy in times of want; whatever the reason, it's a fact.

To make matters worse, when you go off your reduced-calorie diet, you're likely to gain even more weight, and right quick. "A restricted diet causes the body to store fat efficiently," Dr. Fox explains. "When you start eating again, your body is still geared to storing fat." (That old primordial voice again:

A Case for Breastfeeding

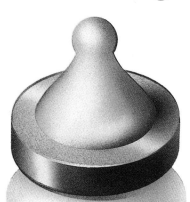

Formula-fed babies, studies have shown, are more prone to be fat than babies fed at the breast. What, you may wonder, is so wrong with having a pudgy baby?

Plenty. For one thing, infancy is a critical time period for the development of fat cells. These will remain with a person for life. Also, fat babies tend to grow into fat children and, later, into fat adults.

Both are good reasons for mothers to breastfeed.

"Hey, food! Better store all the fat I can . . .")

So diets don't work, and some diets can be downright unhealthy and even dangerous.

Weight-loss drugs aren't the answer either. While there are all kinds of drugs available, both prescription and over-the-counter, Dr. Straw states that none has been shown to be effective on a long-term basis, and all of them carry certain risks and potential problems. Various types of radical intervention such as gastrointestinal surgery are also available as means of weight loss, but again Dr. Straw warns that there are dangers; radical intervention should be considered only when a person is so fat that life is endangered and only after consulting a physician.

DO YOU REALLY NEED TO LOSE WEIGHT?

If all of this seems discouraging, start by asking yourself one question: Do I really need to lose weight? "Look at the way the body build of Miss America has changed over the years," points out Dr. Levitsky. "Statistics show that our ideal is getting thinner and thinner. In television commercials and magazine ads, we're bombarded by the image of the super-thin person abundantly enjoying some product. There's a great disparity between the ideal and the actual, and it seems to be growing."

"Lots of people who are only mildly overweight are unhappy because they *think* they should be thinner," says Dr. Piziak.

"Our society fosters the idea that thin is beautiful," adds Dr. Straw, "but is it?" It's worth considering that your desire to lose weight stems from the conflict between what you see in the media and what you see in the mirror. And if that's so, your problem is relatively easy to solve: All you have to do is refuse to accept somebody else's image of what you ought to look like.

That should put some people at ease—but what about the rest of us? At what point do imagination and

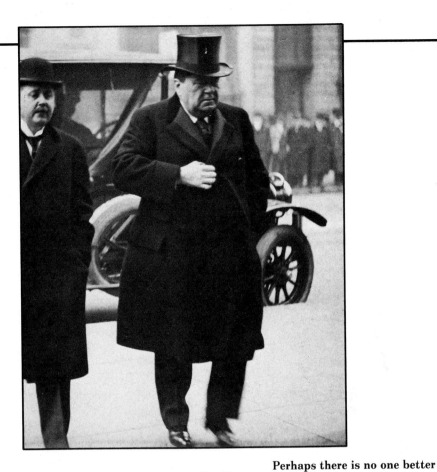

misperception give way to reality? Well, it's indisputable that at some point overweight becomes a serious health problem. The harmful effects of obesity were recorded in antiquity by the Greek physician Hippocrates, who noted an association of overweight with sudden death. Since then, overweight has been linked to a variety of diseases and medical problems.

There are other good reasons to lose weight, too. According to a study of extremely obese men conducted at the Veterans' Administration Wadsworth Hospital Medical Center in Los Angeles, excess weight rendered these people less alert and less mobile, and therefore more vulnerable to accidents. In addition, says Dr. Levitsky, "There's a clear prejudicial atmosphere against fat people. They're discriminated against with respect to employment and promotion and in social interactions. It's irrational and infamous, but it's a fact." Or as Dr. Fox succinctly puts it: "That's the way it is." Even many doctors and counselors hold negative attitudes toward overweight people, reflecting the feelings of society at large, contends Steven P. Kaplan, Ph.D., director of rehabilitation at St.

(continued on page 12)

Perhaps there is no one better to epitomize excess than the turn-of-the-century railroad equipment salesman and bon vivant Diamond Jim Brady. Brady, legend tells us, had a capacity for food that defied belief. Diamond Jim breakfasted on a gallon of orange juice, eggs, cornbread, muffins, flapjacks, chops, fried potatoes and beefsteak. In the late morning, he snacked on 2 or 3 dozen clams and oysters. Lunch was more clams and oysters, 2 or 3 deviled crabs, a brace of broiled lobsters, beef, salad and pie. For afternoon tea he had a heaping plate of seafood washed down by a few bottles of lemon soda (he preferred it to the hard stuff). A typical dinner was 2 or 3 dozen more oysters, ½ dozen crabs, a few bowls of soup, 6 or 7 lobsters, 2 entire ducks, 2 portions of turtle meat, a sirloin steak, vegetables and an assortment of desserts. He capped it all off with a 2-pound box of candy. The tab, by the way, usually went on his expense account. When Brady died at the age of 61 (he had been suffering from stomach problems for 5 years), an autopsy showed he had a stomach 6 times larger than that of an average man.

Problems from Plenty

The world's largest pizza . . . fast food without even having to get out of your car . . . row upon row of restaurants. An abundance of food is literally at our fingertips! It's hard to believe that throughout most of history, one of life's most difficult tasks actually has been getting enough food to survive. In the United States and other Western societies, however, modern agricultural techniques and technological advances have produced a cornucopia of palatable foods. With so much temptation so readily available, overweight may be a natural—though *not* inevitable—consequence.

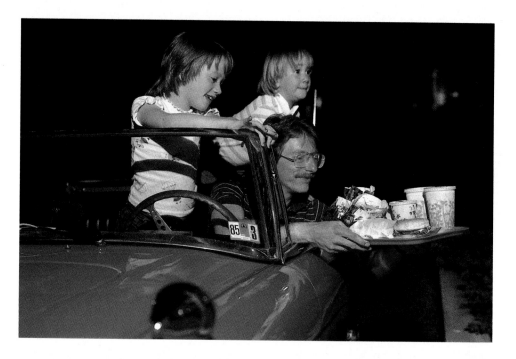

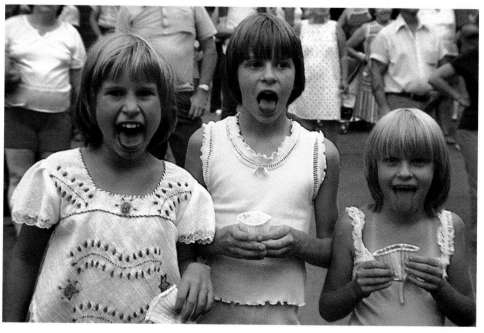

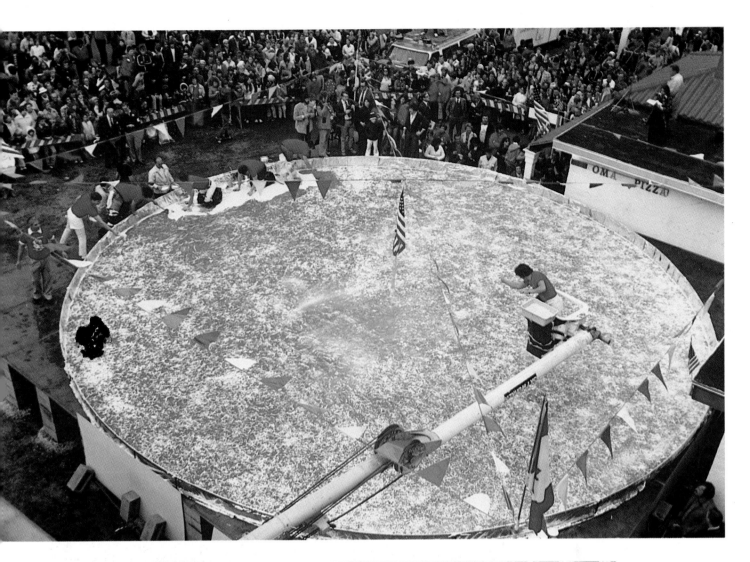

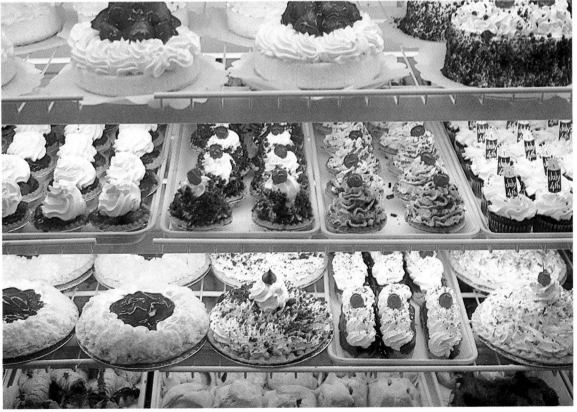

By the volume of fad diet books being sold, it appears that millions of people are looking for a magic formula to help them erase the pounds. In fact, most fad diets are probably doomed to failure because there is no magical means to lose weight.

Some of the most popular diet books are *The Complete Scarsdale Medical Diet*, 7,000,000 copies sold; *The Doctor's Quick Weight Loss Diet*, 5,500,000 copies; *Dr. Atkins' Diet Revolution*, 3,000,000 copies; *The Drinking Man's Diet*, 2,400,000 copies; *The Pritikin Permanent Weight Loss Manual*, 2,000,000 copies; *The Beverly Hills Diet*, 816,500 copies; *The F-Plan Diet*, 110,000 copies; *The Last Chance Diet*, 100,000 copies; and *The Dallas Doctors' Diet*, 8,615 copies.

Vincent Hospital, Green Bay, Wisconsin.

On the positive side of the coin, Dr. Straw points out, "Most successful dieters feel better and gain improved self-esteem." Adds Dr. Kaplan, recalling the 60 pounds he shed and has kept off: "I felt pretty good about it."

AN EASY, GRADUAL WAY TO LOSE WEIGHT

But if civilization is at odds with evolution, diets don't work and drugs and radical intervention are

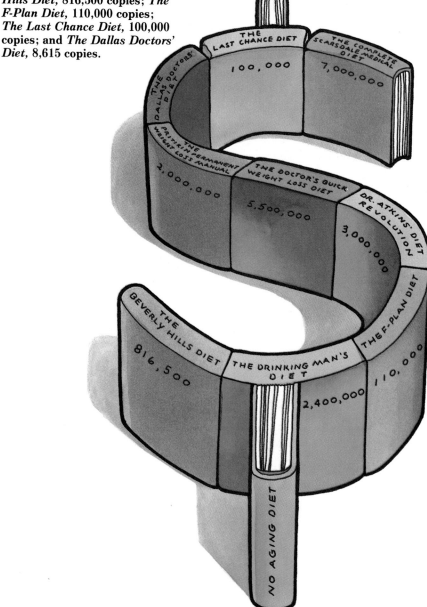

equally to be avoided, what's the solution?

Well, it's really a matter of *solutions,* a lifestyle approach that takes into account all the factors that keep you overweight, and addresses each one with an easy, gradual, no-punishment system. "The answers for most problems in life are not that complicated," Dr. Fox points out. "Take control, make choices; you control your own health."

"The battle of the bulge is not hopeless," adds Dr. Levitsky. "Anyone can lose and maintain a weight loss indefinitely. What is important is a clear, personal reason and determination to lose weight and the realization that a change in body image is what is desired. Concentrate on improving your *life,* not on losing your weight."

In other words, think *energy balance.* "We're overnourished and underexercised," says Dr. Piziak. That means we've got to consider both sides of the equation. So, while diet alone won't achieve permanent weight loss, it *is* an essential ingredient in any weight-loss plan. "Just decreasing fat intake and increasing complex carbohydrates will lead to some weight loss," says Dr. Levitsky. Dr. Fox recommends a diet that's low in fat, moderate (reasonable) in protein and high in complex carbohydrates.

But that's only half the equation. "People who are overweight must diet to lose weight," says Dr. Straw, "but if they don't exercise regularly, they won't be able to maintain that weight loss." Adds Dr. Wadden: "Energy expenditure is just as important as what we eat." Without exercise, in fact, weight control is very difficult, no matter how carefully you watch your diet. Conversely, "weight will drop off automatically as you begin to exercise," insists Dr. Levitsky, "even if intake doesn't change." Here's why.

To begin with, you're burning extra calories while you exercise. In addition, says Dr. Piziak, "regular exercise and body conditioning increase metabolism," and Dr. Stern points out that this effect lasts for hours after you've stopped exercising. What that means is that people who exercise regularly can actually burn up more calories even while *not* exercising than people who don't exercise. Finally, says Dr. Stern, "exercise helps counter the excesses in our diets, and can help avoid weight gain with age."

"We can't go backwards," says Dr. Gutin, another strong advocate of exercise. "We can't get rid of elevators and electric typewriters. I'm not talking about going back to the 1880s. But we can adopt a high-energy lifestyle." That doesn't mean you need to go out and run 5 miles a day. It does mean that you need to find ways to counter the effects of the thousands of small reductions in energy expenditure that cushion our lives—and turn *us* into cushions.

But most of all, what you need is patience. Yes, patience. The battle of the bulge is a war of attrition. "Nobody got fat overnight," says Dr. Levitsky, "and you can't lose weight overnight. There's no such thing as a quick fix. You've got to concentrate on the long run—change your *lifestyle;* nothing short of that will work."

"We want the quick fix," echoes Dr. Fox, "but it doesn't work that way. Rapid weight loss is not the answer. The body resists major changes like that, so you've got to lose weight gradually in order not to upset the system. Weight control isn't an immediate battle; it's a lifelong commitment."

In short, there's no super diet that can help you, no gimmick, no revolutionary technique. So if you're serious about losing weight, make up your mind that you're in it for the long haul.

And if you make up your mind to do that, your prospects for success are really very good—much better than the statistics indicate because the statistics on weight loss are taken from, in Dr. Kaplan's words, "a skewed sampling. People who show up in the medical and psychological literature on obesity are those who ask for help. They're the problem patients, the ones who can't do it on their own. For instance," he continues, again referring to his own successful attempt to lose weight, "I would never have

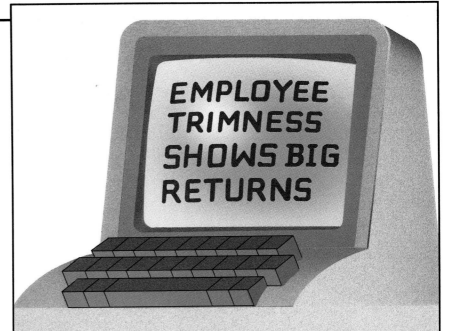

EMPLOYEE TRIMNESS SHOWS BIG RETURNS

Corporate dollars spent on employee weight-control programs can translate into higher corporate profits. That's the conclusion of Lincoln Ekman, Ph.D., of the College of St. Thomas in St. Paul, Minnesota.

Dr. Ekman conducted a study of 32 Minnesota Mutual Life Insurance Company employees who participated in a voluntary weight-control program. The employees attended 1-hour sessions once a week for 12 weeks, during which they learned about nutrition, exercise, relaxation and stress management. During the course of the program, the participants lost an average of 8.7 pounds each.

Dr. Ekman's 1-year follow-up revealed some startling facts. In the year following their weight loss, the participants missed an average of 2.55 fewer work days than the year before. When compared to a control group for the same year, they averaged 3.65 fewer sick days. In terms of days *not* lost to absenteeism, the company's return on its investment in the program ranged between 156 and 363 percent.

shown up in the research because I never asked for help."

"Most people who successfully lose weight do it on their own," agrees Dr. Wadden. They don't join therapeutic weight-loss programs and they don't turn up at the university research clinics. They simply decide to lose weight, find out how to do it, and then *do* it—which is exactly what you're in the process of doing!

Your Real "Ideal" Weight___

It was great news for fat people, the 60 percent of the United States population who weigh more than they should. They weren't overweight anymore. A 5'4" woman with a "medium frame" could tip the scales at 138 pounds— and her weight would be perfect. A 5'9" man with a medium frame could weigh in at 160—and his doctor couldn't say a word about it.

How did a calculator succeed where 500 fad diets failed?

Well, the Metropolitan Life Insurance Company—the folks who put together the standard "ideal weight" charts that most physicians treat as gospel—had decided to revise the ideal weights upward by 5 to 15 percent. And not because the company's president had grown a new set of love handles. They made the change because scientific data show that the death rate is *highest*

among the *thinnest* part of the population.

Or so the statistics *seem* to show. But, says William Castelli, M.D., one of the nation's top experts on who dies for what reasons (a medical science called epidemiology), the statistics lie—until you give them the third degree. Then they tell you that 82 percent of the "thinnest" people are also smokers. And that it's not being skinny that's killing them, it's cancer.

"A scientist from the government's National Heart, Lung and Blood Institute found that lung cancer is a major killer among thin people," explains Dr. Castelli. "And those people are still at risk for the cancer 10 to 15 years after they stop smoking. So an insurance company looking at these deaths might not realize that they are linked to a person's smoking habits, not to

Desirable Weights for Men[1]

Height (in 1-inch heels)	Small frame		Medium frame		Large frame	
	1959	1983	1959	1983	1959	1983
5 ft. 2 in.	112-120	128-134	118-129	131-141	126-141	138-150
5 ft. 3 in.	115-123	130-136	121-133	133-143	129-144	140-153
5 ft. 4 in.	118-126	132-138	124-136	135-145	132-148	142-156
5 ft. 5 in.	121-129	134-140	127-139	137-148	135-152	144-160
5 ft. 6 in.	124-133	136-142	130-143	139-151	138-156	146-164
5 ft. 7 in.	128-137	138-145	134-147	142-154	142-161	149-168
5 ft. 8 in.	132-141	140-148	138-152	145-157	147-166	152-172
5 ft. 9 in.	136-145	142-151	142-156	148-160	151-170	155-176
5 ft. 10 in.	140-150	144-154	146-160	151-163	155-174	158-180
5 ft. 11 in.	144-154	146-157	150-165	154-166	159-179	161-184
6 ft. 0 in.	148-158	149-160	154-170	157-170	164-184	164-188
6 ft. 1 in.	152-162	152-164	158-175	160-174	168-189	168-192
6 ft. 2 in.	156-167	155-168	162-180	164-178	173-194	172-197
6 ft. 3 in.	160-171	158-172	167-185	167-182	178-199	176-202
6 ft. 4 in.	164-175	162-176	172-190	171-187	182-204	181-207

[1] 1959 figures are for men aged 25 and over in "indoor clothing." 1983 figures are for men aged 25-59 in 5 pounds of indoor clothing.

lower body weight."

But Dr. Castelli doesn't think the new weight charts are just wrong. He thinks they're unhealthy, too.

"Today's average American male weighs almost 20 percent more than the weight recommended in Metropolitan's old tables, which were formulated in 1959. And that increase means an increased tendency to heart and circulatory disease, diabetes, high blood pressure and a host of other problems."

In fact, overweight people actually have a higher death rate than nonsmoking thin people. "Studies show that among Seventh-Day Adventists—a religious group that shuns smoking and is leaner than the average American—the men live an average of 6 years and the women 3 years longer than most Americans."

If Dr. Castelli wants to throw out the new Metropolitan Life tables, what does he plan to replace them with? The old ones.

"The 1959 tables show a more realistic weight range than those just revised," he says. But, he adds, women can use the new tables by subtracting 15 percent from the weights; men can use them verbatim—if they use the *women's* weights. "Yet the best way to calculate 'ideal weight,'" says Dr. Castelli, "is to get back to the weight you were in your late teens and early twenties, provided you were not overweight. Being thin is healthy, yes. But it's important to achieve and maintain your 'ideal weight' in a healthy manner."

So, check your ideal weight in the tables below, keeping in mind that it's the 1959 number you'd rather match.

Desirable Weights for Women[1]

Height[2]	Small frame		Medium frame		Large frame	
	1959	1983	1959	1983	1959	1983
4 ft. 10 in.	92-98	102-111	96-107	109-121	104-119	118-131
4 ft. 11 in.	94-101	103-113	98-110	111-123	106-122	120-134
5 ft. 0 in.	96-104	104-115	101-113	113-126	109-125	122-137
5 ft. 1 in.	99-107	106-118	104-116	115-129	112-128	125-140
5 ft. 2 in.	102-110	108-121	107-119	118-132	115-131	128-143
5 ft. 3 in.	105-113	111-124	110-122	121-135	118-134	131-147
5 ft. 4 in.	108-116	114-127	113-126	124-138	121-138	134-151
5 ft. 5 in.	111-119	117-130	116-130	127-141	125-142	137-155
5 ft. 6 in.	114-123	120-133	120-135	130-144	129-146	140-159
5 ft. 7 in.	118-127	123-136	124-139	133-147	133-150	143-163
5 ft. 8 in.	122-131	126-139	128-143	136-150	137-154	146-167
5 ft. 9 in.	126-135	129-142	132-147	139-153	141-158	149-170
5 ft. 10 in.	130-140	132-145	136-151	142-156	145-163	152-173
5 ft. 11 in.	134-144	135-148	140-155	145-159	149-168	155-176
6 ft. 0 in.	138-148	138-151	144-159	148-162	153-173	158-179

[1]1959 figures are for women aged 25 or over in "indoor clothing." 1983 figures are for women aged 25-59 in 3 pounds of indoor clothing.

[2]1959 figures are for women in 2-inch heels. 1983 figures are for women in 1-inch heels.

2

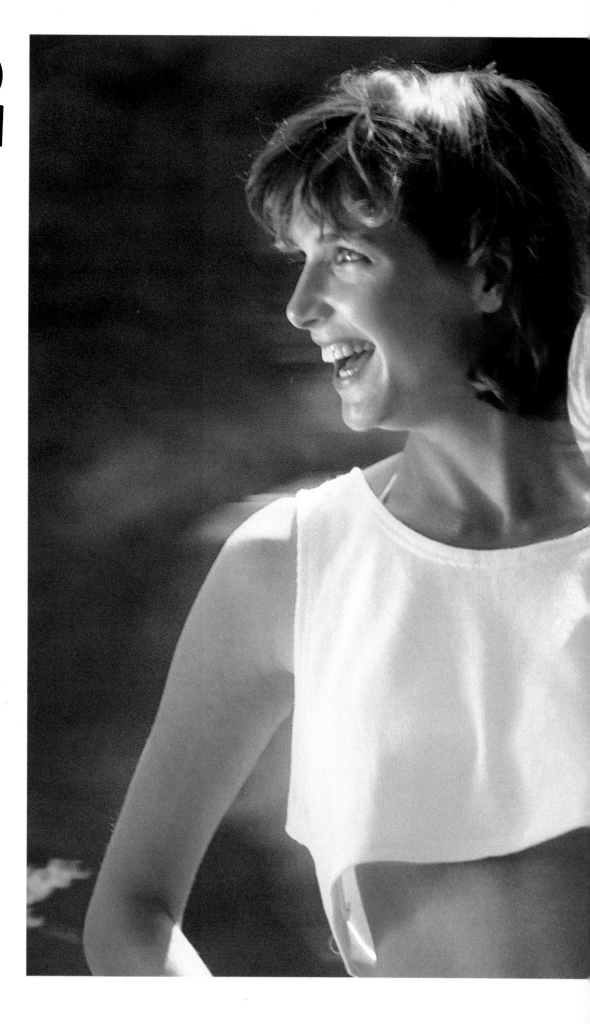

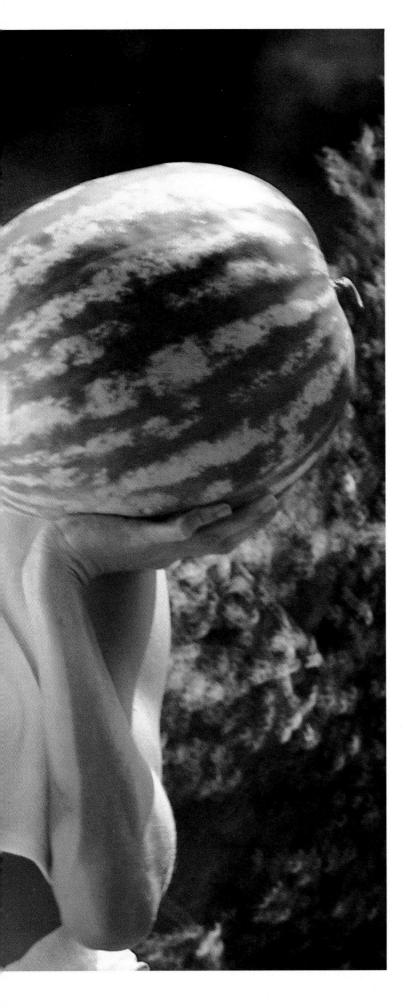

"Slim Foods" for the New You

Forget about "diet foods." There's a vast array of tasty food to get you to your weight-loss goal.

Diet. The word speaks of denial and suffering. The reason is, perhaps, that unappetizing foods have long been promoted as the only way to weight loss. Dietetic "delights" like melba toast, diet soda, black coffee, carrot sticks, baked, unseasoned, skinless chicken, artificial sweeteners that taste like they came off a chemist's shelf and gritty protein drinks have given low-calorie foods a bad reputation. And, in most cases, they deserve it.

Of course, to lose weight you have to burn more calories than you take in. And low-calorie foods like those just mentioned *do* help limit calorie intake—but only as long as you stick to eating just them. It's that restriction that kills most diets. It simply takes too much will power to stick to a dull, lifeless diet. That's why we recommend what we call "slim foods"—foods that fill you up without filling you out. They taste great but keep you from gaining weight. And, best of all, you won't think of them as diet foods.

What are these exciting foods? Well, they're probably already part of your diet, but you just don't think of them as "diet foods." By looking at these foods in a different way, preparing them differently and eating them differently, you can turn your normal diet into a slim-foods gourmet delight. In this chapter we'll show you how.

It's easy to start. Take a mental inventory of your daily menu. Do you eat potatoes? Fish? Vegetables? Grains? Pasta? Chicken? All of these are slim foods and should be part of your weight-loss diet. Yes, there *is* life beyond celery sticks and endless glasses of water!

STAY WITH REAL FOOD AND STILL LOSE WEIGHT

Many people like to sit down to a hearty evening meal of beef, potatoes, cooked vegetables and salad. Often these meat-and-potato folks think that dieting means giving up traditional foods. The thought, however, is wrong. It is a matter of rethinking your meat and potatoes. A generous serving of fatty rib roast, for example, totals 819 calories, but a similar serving of lean rib roast is only 287 calories. That's a 65

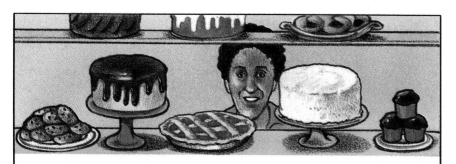

Looking at Food *Can* Make You Fat!

Scientists just may have proven what some people have suspected for a long time: Just looking at food can make them fat.

Judith Rodin, Ph.D., a weight-loss specialist and professor of psychology and psychiatry at Yale University, discovered this after measuring the reactions in a group of formerly fat people to a thick, juicy steak sizzling on a grill in front of them. It was to be their reward after an 18-hour fast. Dr. Rodin took blood samples as they watched the steak cooking.

"Those who were highly responsive to the steak cooking before them had high levels of insulin release," Dr. Rodin says. "Being turned on just by the sight of the food set their metabolic process in motion. Insulin accelerates the intake of fat into the cells, so the more insulin that is secreted, the faster the fat will be stored."

In short, those who drooled over the steak turned more of it into fat than those who didn't. So if the sight of luscious food turns your craving switch to "on," you might want to be somewhat more vigilant in your weight-loss program.

percent drop! So, one way you can cut calories is by always buying lean cuts of beef and other meats.

The same type of thinking applies to the much-maligned potato. The potato itself isn't very fattening. It's how you cook it and what you put on it that makes the spud either the enemy of the dieter or the slim-food eater's best friend. A half cup of potato salad as a side dish with your rib roast equals 182 calories. But ½ cup of mashed potatoes with milk and butter comes to only about 100 calories. Again, a big drop—almost 50 percent. An order of french fries has 75 calories more than a large, tasty baked potato. With a tablespoon of butter the baker will climb 102 calories, but it will fill you up and satisfy you more than the oil-laden french fries.

As you can see, shaving calories has a lot to do with how you prepare the food—not the food itself. It's these kinds of savings (which we'll go into in more detail later in this chapter) that should be applied in all of your meals. It's a lot more pleasing than denial.

COMPLEX CARBOHYDRATES: FILLING, NOT FATTENING

Forget what the fad diet books say. Protein *isn't* the most important part of a diet plan. Actually, only 8 or 9 percent of our daily calories should be protein. Studies have shown that complex carbohydrates—particularly those that are high in fiber—will help you lose more weight, trim off more fat and even feel better. The reason? Complex carbohydrates—unrefined starches such as potatoes, whole grains such as breads, and fruits and vegetables—are high in bulk but low in energy density. A diet rich in these foods results in an overall lower calorie intake and makes you chew longer and feel fuller. Moreover, fiber has the fabulous ability to escort calories out of the body *before* they turn to fat.

A study at the University of Alabama, Birmingham, proved the effectiveness of high-fiber complex carbohydrates in weight loss. Two groups of ten people, both overweight and of normal weight, were allowed to eat unlimited amounts of food at their three meals a day. One group was given a choice of high-fiber complex-carbohydrate foods, including fruits, grains and vegetables. The other group had a choice of high-fat and high-protein foods, like french fries, chocolate cake and fried eggs. Their food intake was measured without their knowledge. After five days, the two groups switched diets. According to questionnaires the people filled out at the end of each day, both diets were filling, tasty and satisfying. But the remarkable results showed that while eating the high-fiber diet, the study participants consumed an average of 50 percent fewer calories than when they ate the high-fat diet. The people on the high-fiber diet were satisfied, ate as much as they liked and still logged an average of only 1,570 calories a day.

One of the most unique things about fiber is that it actually helps reduce the number of calories the body takes in. One specific type of fiber, called pectin, limits the amount of fat that is absorbed in the intestines, according to Luis A. Guerra, M.D., author of *The Bio-Diet*. Citrus fruit rind is about 30 percent pectin; so Dr. Guerra suggests adding part of the citrus rind to your blender when you make fresh juice. Other good sources of pectin include celery, carrots, green beans and cauliflower. No one knows for sure *why* pectin works differently from other fiber, but research shows that it *does* work.

So, just switching from high-fat foods to tasty, high-fiber complex carbohydrates can cut your calorie consumption a great deal. But don't get *complex* carbohydrates confused with *simple* carbohydrates. Simple carbohydrates come from refined foods like sugar and white flour—two things you want to avoid on your diet. Also, you'll find complex carbohydrates in plant foods—never in animal foods.

If you get a hankering for some rich-tasting treats, turn to naturally rich fruits and nuts to satisfy that need. Aileen Ludington, M.D., of the Norwalk Adventist Health Center in California, suggests using

nuts and avocados to fulfill that occasional craving for fatty foods. Both of these foods are high in calories, but the trick is to use them sparingly, in the way you would use a condiment. Dr. Ludington tells people to sprinkle a few nuts on a salad or other dish when they get a craving for fat. And try using a small amount of mashed avocado with lemon instead of mayonnaise on a sandwich. You'll be surprised at how good it tastes.

THE THREE-MEALS-A-DAY WAY

There's another important element in the slim-foods plan that you should put into practice. That's spreading your eating throughout the day. Starving yourself—skipping breakfast and/or lunch—is only counterproductive. Weight-loss specialists agree that people trying to shed pounds should eat three meals a day if they want lasting results. Arnold Andersen, M.D., an eating disorder specialist from Johns Hopkins Medical School in Baltimore, says that a dieter "should eat according to his or her appetite, and avoid sugars and fats." He says that three meals a day is the best way to do that.

And for those iron-willed few who can limit themselves to one meal a day—even they may have trouble shedding pounds. The reason is that eating all your calories at one time encourages more weight gain than spreading the calories throughout the day. A study of mice proved this point. "Though there are no studies that document the same effect in humans, I find no reason to disagree with the study," says Dr. Andersen. "Conventional wisdom would show that the same thing applies to humans."

The same wisdom also tells you that dieting doesn't have to be a chore. All kinds of foods you used to deprive yourself of on other diets can be enjoyed on your weight-loss plan. On the next few pages, we'll show you how to buy and prepare certain foods in ways that won't make you feel deprived. In no time at all you'll be well on your way to a slender and healthy body.

Foods with a False Reputation

There are a lot of good foods around taking a bum rap for being high in calories (and bad for you) when they're really not. The truth is that they give you a lot of bulk for the calories consumed. Some examples:
- Baked potato (145 calories)
- Spaghetti (155 per cup)
- Bean soup (116 per cup)
- Bran muffins (104 each)
- Tomato sauce (45 per ½ cup)
- Chicken noodle soup (75 per cup)
- Brown rice (116 per ½ cup)
- Popcorn (23 per cup)

On the other hand, there are foods that are passed off as low calorie when they really pack a punch. Eat these sparingly.
- Granola (298 per ½ cup)
- Fruit yogurt (225 per cup)
- Margarine (102 per tablespoon)
- Dried apricots (269 per 4 ounces)
- White wine (80 per 3½ ounces)
- Raisins (248 per ½ cup)

The Clever Cook's Kitchen

Food is tempting. Everybody knows that. But did it ever occur to you that the place you keep your food—namely, the kitchen— could be tempting you, too?

Take a look around your kitchen. The cookie jar in the corner is no dieter's friend. How often do the wrong hands slip into it at your house? Those canisters of sugar, flour and cocoa that you stare at every morning over your coffee cup almost beg you to "turn me into homemade cookies." And guess who ends up eating them?

Everyone loves a kitchen. It's a place to feel comfortable and at home, not a place to set you up for impulse eating. So get rid of the items and tempting kitchen devices that are convenient only for gaining weight. Give them away to slim friends—your cookie jar, sugar bowl, candy dishes and cake savers. Or at least stash them away in a place where you'll need a stepladder just to see them!

Then replace them with some of the items pictured here in our version of the clever cook's kitchen. You don't need to run out and spend all your money on new equipment. You probably already have some of the items; buy the others gradually. Before you know it, you'll have a new kitchen to go along with your new outlook on eating. These tools will make your slim-foods cooking a breeze—almost as easy as slipping on your new, slim clothes.

1. Hot-air popcorn popper—No oil goes into this electric popcorn maker, which can turn out a hot, wholesome and low-calorie snack in a matter of minutes. And it takes up a lot less room than a can of pretzels or potato chips!

2. Blender—Its multifaceted function makes it only practical to have on hand, especially when it comes to pureeing vegetables or soups or whipping up low-calorie drinks.

3. Bouquets garni—Special blends of spices and herbs can turn the ordinary dish into the extraordinary. Make your own blends, wrap them in cheesecloth and keep them in a canister (like the one that used to hold the sugar).

4. Bowl of fruit—You can put this where the cookie jar used to be. If your hand automatically goes in that direction when you're hungry, you'll end up with something nutritious and low in calories to munch on.

5. Garlic braid—No, it's not silly to keep plenty of garlic on hand. In addition to its ability to perk up a bland dish, garlic has amazing health benefits. A braid has an advantage over the single bulbs you buy in the supermarket because the braids are picked at the peak of ripeness to ensure premium quality. Its looks will add charm to your kitchen.

6. Slow cooker—The leanest cuts of meat often require the longest cooking. A slow cooker is the device to use when you don't have a few hours to spare tending to the stove. With a slow cooker you add the ingredients, plug it in and leave for work or shopping. When you get home, the meal is done.

7. Double boiler—Yes, this utensil is good for more than melting chocolate. It helps warm up leftovers (like potatoes, vegetables or meat casseroles) without butter or oil. It also is handy in making the lighter sauces that are part of the clever cook's repertoire.

8. Egg coddler—Remember when Grandma turned out coddled eggs for you for Sunday breakfast? Coddled eggs are a great alternative to eggs fried or scrambled with fat. And they're a lot easier to prepare than poached.

9. Electric juicer—Anyone who's ever tasted freshly squeezed orange juice knows what a wonderful device a juicer is. But its importance to the clever cook goes beyond great taste. By squeezing your own fruit juices you'll retain a bit of the all-important fiber that is strained out of some commercial varieties.

10. Fish poacher—For anyone but the true fish lover, this piece of equipment is indeed extravagant. But if you catch your own fish or live near the water and buy fish fresh and whole, you might want to consider buying a poacher and enjoying your fish the way the Europeans do—delicately cooked with herbs and vegetables in a poaching liquid.

11. Food processor—This handy device can do everything a blender can do and more. It cuts, chops, grates and juliennes vegetables within seconds. Of course, it uses up less calories than the manual method does, but some claim its fine chopping action releases juices, particularly from onions, which reduce the need for butter or oil in sauteing.

12. Grains and legumes—Empty your canisters of sugars and refined flours and refill them with a variety of grains. Split peas, millet and whole wheat pasta make up the dried-foods pantry in this kitchen.

13. Fresh herbs—To make the most of your slim-foods cooking, keep a supply of fresh herbs on your kitchen windowsill. Dried just can't match the taste of, say, fresh basil in a summer tomato salad, or the aroma of fresh tarragon in a light brown sauce.

14. Mortar and pestle—Buying ingredients in their natural form is the way of the wise cook. That's why a mortar and pestle is an important tool in the clever cook's kitchen. It's great for grinding herbs, spices, nuts and seeds.

15. Nonstick pans—Today they come in all sizes and shapes and price ranges. The advantage? They allow you to saute without the addition of *any* fat. Every weight watcher should have at least one.

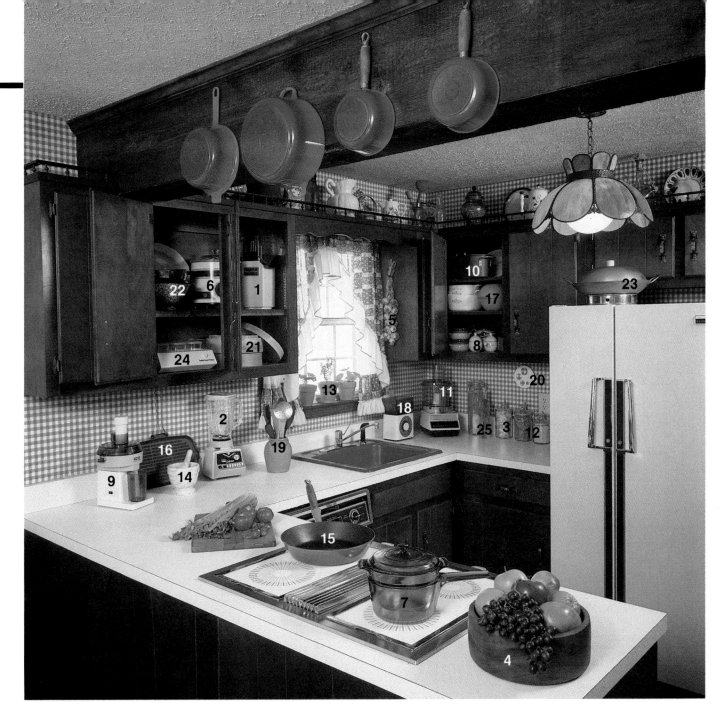

16. Ridged cast-iron skillet—No one wants to give up hamburgers or grilled cheese sandwiches forever. So for those occasional times you do indulge in something fried or grilled, make it in a ridged pan. The ridges help capture excess fat and keep it *off* your food.

17. Clay cooker—Another utensil perhaps only the serious cook can appreciate, the clay cooker allows meats to simmer slowly in their own juices, making the use of extra fats, sauces or broths unnecessary.

18. Scale—Is that really a 3-ounce portion you're serving yourself? When in doubt, lay it out—on your handy kitchen food scale.

19. Skimmers and wooden spoons—A set of each should be in your utensil bowl. Skimmers are just what they seem—they skim the fat off soups and stew. Wooden spoons are essential when using nonstick pans.

20. Spaghetti measurer—How many times have you made spaghetti and wound up with enough to wind around your kitchen—twice? This inexpensive little device guarantees you'll cook the right amount.

21. Steamer—Although you needn't buy the Oriental bamboo variety, a steamer should be part of every kitchen. It is perfect for making vegetables to perfection—*al dente.*

22. Strainer—You'll want to have one of these for rinsing all the fresh fruits and vegetables you'll have on hand.

23. Wok—Stir-fry is a great way to cook. While a little fat is required, you don't need nearly the amount that is required for pan frying. And as your wok gets seasoned with use, you'll find you can get away with using less and less.

24. Yogurt maker—Why buy it when you can make it, especially when you can make it better with less calories.

25. Vinegar—That's right, no oil. Just vinegar. Vinegar can stand alone quite well on a salad.

Cooking It Right

Lose Weight— Tastefully

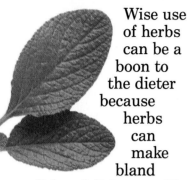

Wise use of herbs can be a boon to the dieter because herbs can make bland dishes delicious—without extra calories. For instance, fish poached in a stock flavored with basil, tarragon and bay leaf is a tasty alternative to fish poached in water or weak chicken broth. Dill, chives and curry can add extra flavor to egg dishes like omelets and frittatas.

Most foods, particularly meats, fish, poultry, and vegetable and rice dishes, take well to herbs. So don't be afraid to use them. Experiment by mixing 2 or more herbs in one dish. Good all-purpose herbs to begin exploring with are basil, oregano, thyme, tarragon and parsley.

One of the most important secrets to successful dieting is learning how to prepare food properly. An innocent low-calorie chicken breast can turn into a dieter's greasy terror if it is coated with bread crumbs and deep fried. A fairly good cut of roast beef will become a calorie-laden nightmare if it is covered with gravy made from fatty drippings. The object of most slim-foods cooking methods is to reduce the fat content of foods while retaining their precious nutrients.

The first step is to get rid of as much fat as you can before cooking the food. That means starting your slim-foods cooking at the grocery store. First, buy lean cuts of meats, but don't buy them too often. Instead, rely on fish and chicken, which are naturally lower in calories. White chicken meat, by the way, is lower than dark—and calories and fat can be further reduced by removing the skin.

In addition to making poultry and fish in place of meat, consider healthful, satisfying meat substitutes such as legumes. This group of vegetables, including black beans, lentils, split peas and others, have a chewy, satisfying texture.

Along with rethinking the meat entree, consider adjusting your side dishes. Serve potatoes baked, sprinkled with chives or herbs in place of butter. Turn to whole wheat pasta or pasta made from spinach or other vegetables instead of the usual white pasta. Try whole grain breads in place of white bread. They're more nutritious and *much* more filling.

When preparing desserts, including baked goods, reduce the sugar called for in recipes by one-half. This calls for a little experience and experimenting by the cook. You also can substitute fructose for sugar in recipes. Using two-thirds the amount called for in the recipe achieves the same level of sweetness. Also consider using fresh fruits in place of sugary desserts. These methods reduce calories while still meeting the needs of your sweet tooth.

Finally, buy low-fat dairy products. Skim and low-fat milk, low-fat yogurt, farmer's cheese,

mozzarella and low-fat cottage cheese are good. And don't be fooled by margarine. Most margarines contain the same number of calories as butter.

Once you get the food home, there are a number of ways to keep the calories way down and the good taste up. Always look at your foods with an eye toward how many calories you can cut out.

One of the biggest problems for dieters is giving up sauces and gravies. Joe Durocher, Ph.D., a chef and a professor at New York University, says the professional secret to making good gravy is to skim the fat from the pan before the gravy is made. "Deglaze the drippings that are left—this is where all the flavor is—with water or bouillon. Then thicken the liquid with cornstarch or flour and water instead of a roux (flour and butter paste)." This gravy is lower in calories and tastes better than the greasy-spoon variety.

When cooking fatty meat, first trim it of all its fat and then braise it in bouillon or water. (In braising, you cook meat in liquid in a closed container.) The longer you cook it, the more fat will seep into the braising liquid. You can use this to your advantage. For example, if you braise the meat the day before and then refrigerate it, the fat will harden on the surface of the broth. You then can remove it with a spoon. The same works for soups and stews.

It's easy to save calories in sauteing, too. For example, if the recipe calls for a tablespoon of butter or oil, use half. Better yet, don't use any fat at all. Try sauteing in chicken or beef stock. You can freeze stock in ice cube trays and use it as needed, as you would butter. Or you could try lecithin-based spray to keep the food from sticking. Or use a nonstick pan. These pans have been greatly improved over the years and are great because with many foods, no oil at all is necessary.

Also, there's no need to throw out your recipes that call for deep frying. Baking can make the dish taste just as good.

The Best (and Worst) Cooking Methods

When it comes to cutting calories and fat, some methods of cooking definitely stand out over others. Here's our glossary of cooking methods with some calorie-cutting tips.

 Baking

Marinate with tea or juice, not oil. Always cover the pan to keep the food moist. An ideal method for fish, squash, potatoes and loaves.

 Boiling

What you gain in reduced calories using this method can be offset by lost nutrients. But you can avoid this by boiling potatoes in their skins and vegetables in boilable plastic bags.

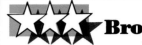 **Broiling**

Don't use extra butter or oil. Use juice or water—not wine—if making a sauce. This method is good for meats and fish fillets.

 Deep Frying

Foods cooked by this method really gobble up the calories in fat. It's best to avoid it altogether. If you do deep fry, you can cut the fat somewhat by draining the food well when it comes out of the fryer.

 Fireplace Cooking

This method, whether used indoors or out, is ideal for stews or soups that need long cooking. Make sure you keep skimming off excess fat during cooking. Also, don't use added fat or oil—you don't need it.

 Outdoor Grilling

The marinades and sauces commonly used in outdoor grilling tend to be high in calories. Avoid oil-based marinades. The healthiest and leanest way is to grill the food plain and wrapped in foil to keep it moist.

 Pan Frying

This method also offers you unwanted fat. But you can cut back by using spray coatings or nonstick pans. Also, avoid the breading that's often called for in pan-frying recipes.

 Poaching

This method is hard to match. Unfortunately, a lot of people don't realize that it's ideal for more than eggs. It's often the tastiest—and leanest—way to prepare fish. Season the poaching liquid with herbs for extra flavor.

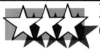 **Pressure Cooking**

Don't add any fat during cooking. Chill and skim off any fat when making stews. Also ideal for dried beans, vegetables, grains and soups.

 Roasting

This method is most often used for beef, pork, veal or poultry roasts. Trim the meat well before roasting and always set the roast on a rack so the fat can run off, not around, the meat.

 Sauteing

This method is often used for onions, mushrooms and peppers and thinly cut chicken or veal fillets. You can cut back on the fat by substituting chicken broth for the oil.

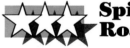 **Spit Roasting**

Another slow-cooking method that allows the meat to expel much of its fat. Don't coat with high-calorie sauces. Rather, marinate the meats in their own juices.

 Steaming

A great way to cook vegetables while keeping the nutrients in. Always use a steaming basket and never use butter. You'll find the food doesn't really need it.

 Stewing

Also known as braising, this method is ideal because the slow cooking allows the meat to give off its fat. You can then get rid of the fat by chilling the stew and skimming it off.

 Stir-Frying

Good for vegetables, beef and chicken. You don't need a lot of fat with this method. By adding a little water or stock you can keep the food moist.

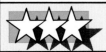 Excellent   Good   Poor

23

Nutritious Slim Foods

S ome diets advise you to stick to one low-calorie food—like grapefruit—for a long period of time. Unfortunately, these diets deprive you of precious nutrients, and what good is being slim if you are also unhealthy? The foods pictured here provide a bounty of nutrients in low-calorie packages. Try them all. The more variety you have in your diet, the more chance you have of coming out a healthy winner in your get-slim diet plan.

For 30 Calories per Serving, or Less . . .

. . . you can get broccoli, and it would be hard to find any food with more nutrition per calorie; carrots, an outstanding source of vitamin A; asparagus and spinach, great providers of vitamins A and C; mung beans, just brimming with minerals; raw mushrooms, a good bet for B's and potassium; and other nutrition-plus foods like green peppers, onions, wheat germ, kale and tomatoes. Put them all together for a super-nutritious salad at a low-calorie price.

For 100 Calories per Serving, or Less . . .

. . . you can have corn on the cob, a nice source of niacin; peas, which will give you plenty of thiamine (vitamin B_1), niacin, protein and iron; acorn squash, a tasty treat that gives you a lot of vitamin C, pantothenate and potassium for a small number of calories; cantaloupe, an outstanding source of vitamins A and C; brussels sprouts, high in B_6 and pantothenate; plus other sweet-tasting things like apricots, mangoes and blackberries.

For 200 Calories per Serving, or Less . . .

. . . you can have meat and nutrition, too. You'll find plenty of protein in sirloin and round steak and they're an important source of B_{12}. Beef liver is a great source of vitamins A and C and the B vitamins. White meat chicken is super-filled with niacin. Salmon is outstanding in B vitamins and also contains plenty of calcium (if you eat the bones). And, yes, you can have navy beans, which are a great way to get protein and fiber. Lima beans are a good source of vitamin C.

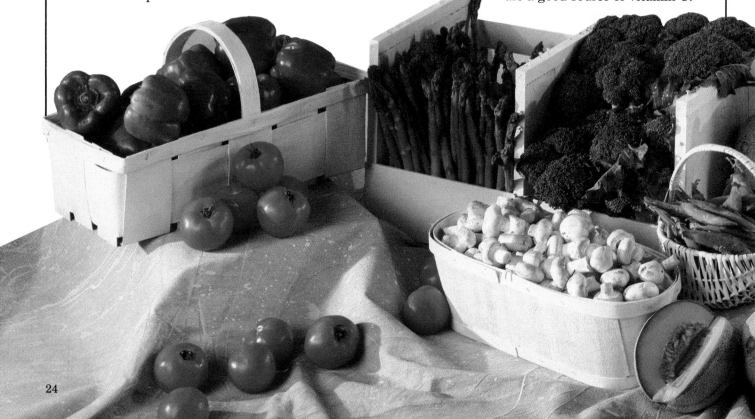

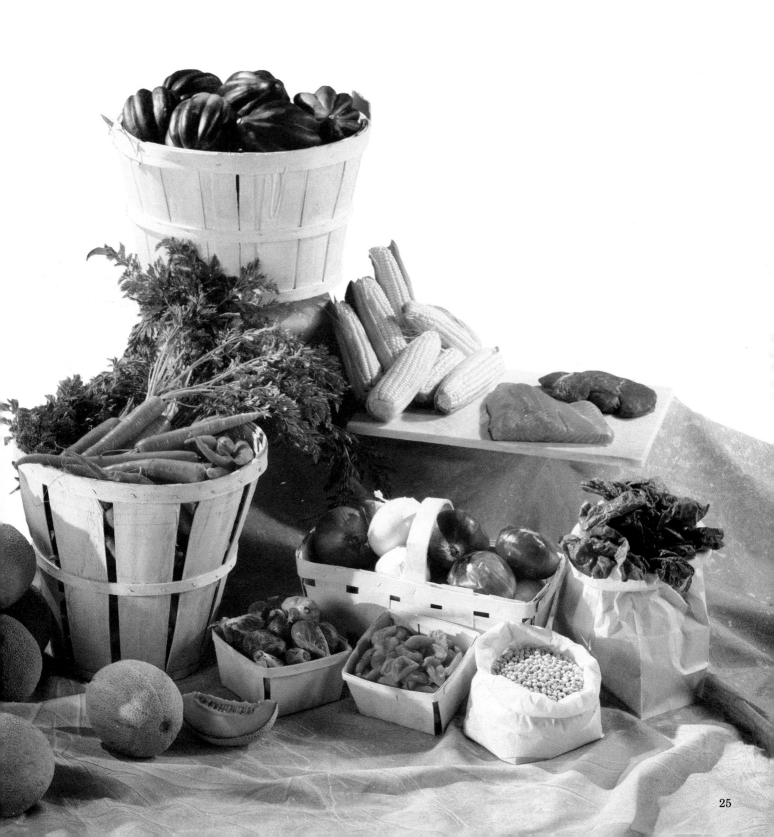

Meat Buyer's Guide

If you are an avid meat eater and want to lose weight, you'll be glad to know that you don't have to scratch roasts, chops, steaks and drumsticks off your menu. While adding more fresh fruits, grains and vegetables to your diet is a necessary part of any slim-foods plan, you can continue to enjoy your favorite meats. In fact, beef, poultry, pork and lamb are all healthy slim foods; you just have to know which cuts to pick. Stick with lean meat and you won't go wrong. Meat is a good part of any diet because it is very nutritious, supplying high amounts of protein and important vitamins and minerals like iron and B vitamins. Use the guides on these pages when you make up your shopping list. Just remember, all calorie counts listed are for 3-ounce servings, an amount that will satisfy but not stuff you.

The Choicest Cuts

Next time you're hankering for a piece of meat, but want to stay on the light side of the calorie chart, stick with the meats suggested below. Remember, these figures for the top 10 are for poultry without the skin and bone and lean, trimmed, good grade meat.

Meat	Calories per 3-oz. Serving	Percent of Calories from Fat
Turkey breast	115	4.9
Turkey leg	135	21.5
Turkey wing	139	19.1
Chicken breast	140	19.5
Chicken drumstick	147	29.6
Heel of round	148	25.9
Round steak	149	22.2
Beef foreshank	150	24.6
Beef hindshank	150	24.6
Chuck steak	152	26.1

Poultry

When it comes to low-calorie food, poultry is nothing to squawk at. It is one of the best all-around diet foods—though you have to watch out for a few high-fat cuts—and it's relatively inexpensive and easy to prepare. There are a few secrets to choosing and preparing your birds, however. A large source of calories in poultry is the skin, and the fat that lies just underneath. Removing the skin and fat *before* you cook the bird will reduce the fat content by almost half. For example, one whole uncooked chicken breast has 87 percent more fat than a breast with the skin removed. A whole drumstick has 61 percent more fat than a skinless drumstick. A trimmed, lean thigh has 74 percent less fat than a whole thigh. So, remove the skin and remember this tip: Thighs are highest in calories to start with, because they have more fat, and breasts are lowest.

The type of bird you choose to cook also makes a difference in the calories you consume. According to Linda Posati, a nutritionist with the United States Department of Agriculture (USDA), "Turkey is the leanest poultry you can buy." She also says that the younger the turkey, the better: "Hens and toms are larger and much higher in fat and calories than young turkeys." The USDA rates the varying types of poultry by fat content as follows (fig-

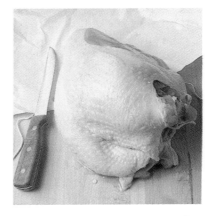

ures are per 100 grams, or 3½ ounces, of a whole bird, minus the neck and giblets): Chicken, 15.06 grams with skin but only 3.08 grams without; turkey, 8.02 with skin, but only 2.86 without; duck, 39.34 with skin but only 5.95 without; goose, 33.62 with skin but only 7.13 without.

Judging from these figures, it might be wise to save duck and goose for special occasions. Stick to chicken and turkey, and make no bones about removing the skin.

Beef

Beef is by far the most popular meat in America, and also the one blamed most often for weight gain. Well, in some ways beef deserves its bad reputation; many cuts *are* fattening. But if you avoid high-calorie, high-fat cuts of beef, there is no reason why steaks and roasts can't be a part of your slim-foods diet. First, as with all meat, you should learn to trim any extra fat from the beef you buy.

If you stick with lean meats, you won't feel deprived. Versatile round steak has only 162 calories per serving, about the same as a chuck steak. The fat can be easily trimmed from either of these. Flank steak, which is usually lean when purchased, can be tenderized with a marinade and broiled or grilled. It contains only 167 calories.

If you feel like celebrating with a steak dinner, don't let your diet spoil the occasion. Try a sirloin steak, with 204 calories per serving, or a T-bone or porterhouse, which have about 190 calories per serving.

The best advice is to avoid any roasts or

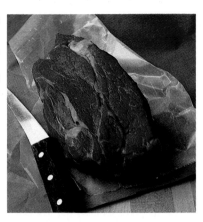

steaks that are well marbled or pocked with fatty areas.

Avoid ribs —the meat is usually connected to the bone by a healthy portion of fat. Club steak and rib roasts are also high in fat and calories. Some of the worst offenders are chuck rib roast, with 321 calories per serving, and corned beef, which will add 317 calories to your frame.

Finally, don't gravitate toward the cheaper ground beef; it is usually highest in fat. Leaner beef costs more, but doesn't shrink as much during cooking and is far lower in calories.

Pork

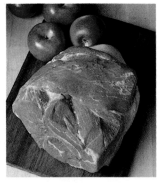

Pork producers have responded to the nation's desire for low-calorie foods by breeding animals that are leaner. The results are encouraging for dieters: Pork averages only 198 calories per serving. The best all-around cut of pork in terms of calories is a lightly cured ham, which weighs in at 140 calories per serving. However, ham does have its drawbacks. For one, it's high in salt, which can make you retain water. So it's best to use such cuts sparingly, if at all. Rather, you might want to go for a fresh ham—also low in calories at 188 per serving—which has much less salt. You should also consider a loin cut of pork, at 204 calories per serving. Its tenderloin is a mere 141 calories!

Lamb

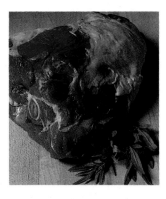

Because of its expense, lamb is seen by many Americans as a special treat served on rare occasions. But the expense is well worth it if it's lean and low-calorie meat that you're after. An average serving costs only 150 calories. Some cuts are better than others, of course, and leg of lamb is at the top. A cooked 3-ounce portion will add only 156 calories to your energy supply. Lamb shank, which can be cooked in many different ways, has only 153 calories per serving. And an elegant portion of rack of lamb contains only 197 calories. In fact, lamb is an all-around good meat for weight-conscious people. The cut that weighs in with the most calories—arm chops—still has only 237 per serving.

The Cheese Lover's Guide

It's true that cheese is the central ingredient in many calorie-laden dishes like souffles, quiches, pizza and casseroles. But that doesn't mean you have to give it up! For one thing, cheese is good for you. It's a rich source of protein and calcium and it also has a good supply of vitamin A and B vitamins, especially riboflavin (vitamin B_2).

The secret to having your cheese and a nice waistline, too, is to choose your cheese with care. For daily fare, try to pick cheeses that are high in the good things (like protein and calcium) and low in the bad things (like fat and salt).

Because it's high in fat, cheese packs a lot of calories into a small space. That isn't a problem if you eat your cheese in 1-ounce servings (about a 2-inch cube). But if you like thick cheese sandwiches or can munch endlessly on cheese hors d'oeuvres, be aware that the calories add up quickly.

You can figure that most cheeses will give you around 100 calories per ounce. Brie, Limburger, Tilsit, provolone, blue cheese, brick cheese, Muenster and Roquefort are all within 10 calories of the 100-calorie mark. Cottage cheese, the dieter's staple, comes out on the bottom of the calorie scale, at a meager 25 calories per ounce for 2 percent fat cottage cheese and 29 calories for regular, so you're not saving that many calories by opting for the low-fat version. On the other hand, you don't usually eat just an ounce of cottage cheese. A normal serving is around 4 ounces, which brings the total back to that 100-calorie neighborhood.

There are a few other particularly low-calorie cheeses, like part-skim mozzarella (72 calories per ounce) and Neufchatel (74 calories). The creamier cheeses that are high in fat are also, of course, higher in calories. Gjetost, a Norwegian cheese, weighs in at a hefty 132 calories per ounce.

A good rule of thumb to keep in mind is that generally the harder cheeses, like cheddar and Swiss, are higher in calories than the soft cheeses. "This is because harder cheeses are aged longer," says Jane Holmes, a vice president for the American Dairy Association. For example, cheddar cheese is aged for 4 to 12 months, while cottage cheese must be consumed soon after it is made. "Aging cuts the amount of liquid, concentrating the cheese

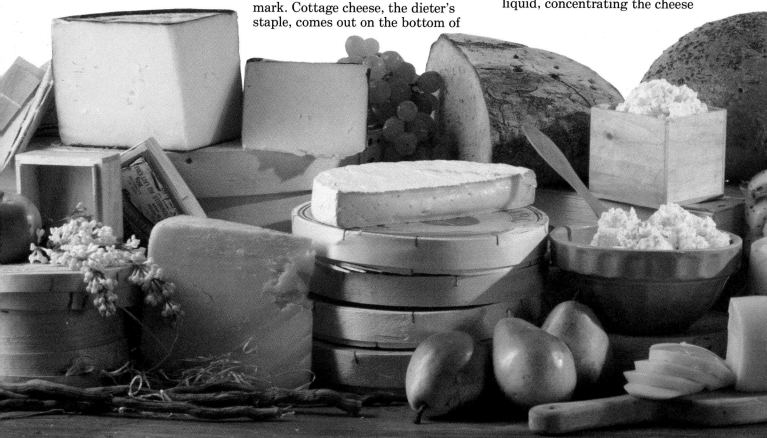

and—of course—the calories," says Ms. Holmes. An exception to this rule, she points out, would be hard cheeses like Parmesan and Romano, which are often used only sparingly as seasonings. But, generally, remember to eat harder cheeses in moderation.

BE INNOVATIVE

Unfortunately, many of the cheeses you can eat more liberally—cottage cheese is the most obvious example—can get boring after a while if you just eat them plain. But there are scores of innovative ways you can use such cheeses to your taste advantage.

Blend cottage cheese or a little ricotta into potato or chicken salad to cut back on mayonnaise. Use cottage cheese instead of ricotta in lasagna (you'll save almost half the calories), or use them together. Spread cottage cheese on toast in the morning instead of using butter. If you mix it with a little apple butter, you'll have a good-tasting, low-calorie spread.

Calories at a Glance

Want to get the most cheese for the least calories? Then start with farmer's cheese, which weighs in at only 43 calories per ounce. The table below gives you a weight watcher's account of the more popular cheeses in ascending caloric order. Make your selection wisely.

Cheese	Portion	Calories	Percent of Calories from Fat
Farmer's cheese	1 oz.	43	58.0
Cottage cheese, dry curd	½ cup	62	4.4
Mozzarella, part skim	1 oz.	72	55.1
Neufchatel	1 oz.	74	78.9
Feta cheese	1 oz.	75	70.7
Mozzarella	1 oz.	80	67.2
Cottage cheese, 1% low fat	½ cup	82	12.3
Camembert	1 oz.	85	71.2
Limburger	1 oz.	93	73.0
Brie	1 oz.	95	72.6
Cream cheese	1 oz.	99	87.8
Blue cheese	1 oz.	100	71.6
Cottage cheese, 2% low fat	½ cup	102	18.9
Brick cheese	1 oz.	105	70.4
Roquefort	1 oz.	105	72.8
American	1 oz.	106	73.5
Swiss	1 oz.	107	63.9
Armenian string cheese	1 oz.	108	66.5
Cottage cheese, creamed	½ cup	109	38.4
Parmesan, hard	1 oz.	111	58.0
Cheddar	1 oz.	114	72.5
Ricotta, part skim	½ cup	171	50.4

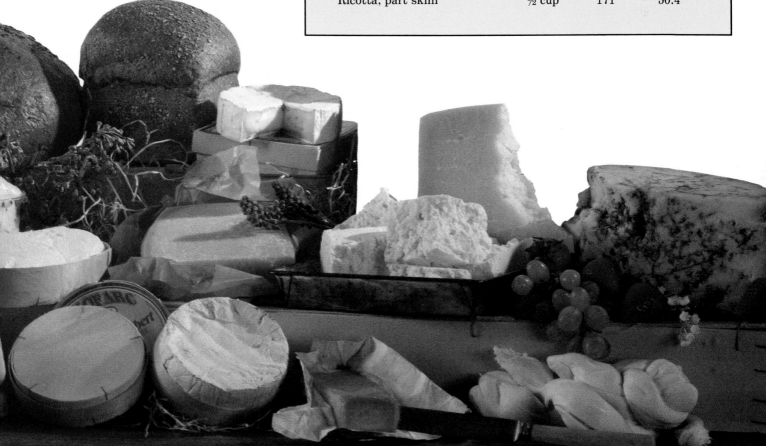

Snacks and Desserts

If you slink away from diets out of fear that you won't be able to enjoy occasional snacks and desserts, take heart. Our seasoned chefs have found several ways for you to partake of such treats and still avoid the extra padding around your legs, stomach and derriere that comes with a diet of hot-fudge sundaes, ice cream and cookies.

These delicious, nutritious, *low-calorie* snacks are so delightful that you'll soon forget that you are trying to lose weight. Just remember that even these aren't the total answer to your weight problem. Eat them in moderation, as you would any other food.

Fruit Kabobs with Yogurt Sauce

Makes 30 snacks (about 45 calories each)

¼ fresh pineapple, cut into 30 chunks
¾ cup green seedless grapes (about 30 grapes)
2 navel oranges, peeled and sectioned
1 cup strawberries, halved
8 ounces Swiss, cheddar or Monterey Jack cheese, cubed
Orange Yogurt Sauce

Place three pieces of any combination of fruit and cheese on a toothpick. Place attractively on a platter or tray. Serve with orange yogurt sauce.

ORANGE YOGURT SAUCE

1 cup yogurt
2 tablespoons maple syrup or honey
2 tablespoons grated orange rind

Place the ingredients in a medium bowl and mix until thoroughly combined. Refrigerate until ready to use. (This recipe makes 1¼ cups of sauce with 14 calories per tablespoon.)

Cheese Popcorn

Makes 10 cups (48 calories each)

1 tablespoon grated Romano cheese
1 tablespoon grated Parmesan cheese
1 teaspoon hot chili powder
10 cups popped corn
2 tablespoons butter, melted

Mix the cheeses and chili powder together in a small bowl. Place the popcorn in a large bowl. Drizzle butter over popcorn and toss. Sprinkle with cheese mixture and toss until thoroughly combined.

Pickled Cauliflower

Makes 16 servings (about 25 calories each)

1 quart white wine vinegar or cider vinegar
2 tablespoons mustard seeds
½ cup honey
⅛ teaspoon turmeric
8 whole cloves
4 sticks cinnamon
2 medium heads cauliflower

Place all ingredients except the cauliflower in a 1½- to 2-quart saucepan. Bring to a boil, then reduce heat and simmer for 15 minutes.

Meanwhile, wash the cauliflower, cut away all leaves and break into florets. Blanch in boiling water for 2 minutes. Drain the florets and put them into jars, then pour the hot liquid and spices over them. Cover and refrigerate. The cauliflower will keep for several weeks.

Blueberry Pudding

Makes 8 servings (98 calories each)

2 cups low-fat cottage cheese
1 cup yogurt
2 tablespoons honey
3 tablespoons lemon juice
2 cups blueberries, washed and drained

Place the cottage cheese in a blender and blend, then add remaining ingredients and mix well. Chill before serving.

Variation: Use strawberries, raspberries or sliced peaches, either instead of the blueberries or in combination with them. Place the pudding in a pie plate lined with granola or in a prepared baked pie crust.

Whole Wheat Sponge Cake

Makes 12 servings (116 calories each)

6 eggs, separated
1 teaspoon vanilla extract
½ cup honey, warmed
1 tablespoon lemon juice
1 teaspoon grated lemon rind
1 cup whole wheat flour

Cut waxed paper to fit the bottom of a 9-inch tube pan. Butter the bottom of the pan; place waxed paper on the bottom, then butter the waxed paper. Do not grease the sides of the pan.

Place the egg whites and vanilla in a medium bowl. Using an electric mixer, beat until they are very stiff. Continue beating, and add the honey in a slow, thin stream. Beat until the mixture is stiff and forms peaks.

Combine the lemon juice and rind and egg yolks in a medium bowl. Then fold one-fourth of the egg whites thoroughly into the yolks, using a wire whisk to stir, not beat, the eggs. Pour this mixture over the remaining egg whites and sprinkle the flour on top. Gently fold all the ingredients together, taking care to incorporate all the flour, yet not lose too much air from the egg whites.

Pour or spoon the batter into the prepared pan and bake in a preheated 350°F oven for 20 to 30 minutes. When the cake is golden brown and springy to the touch, and the sides begin to pull away from the pan, invert the pan on a cooling rack immediately. Let cool for 10 minutes, then loosen the sides of the cake with a knife and remove from pan. Remove the waxed paper and set cake on rack until cool.

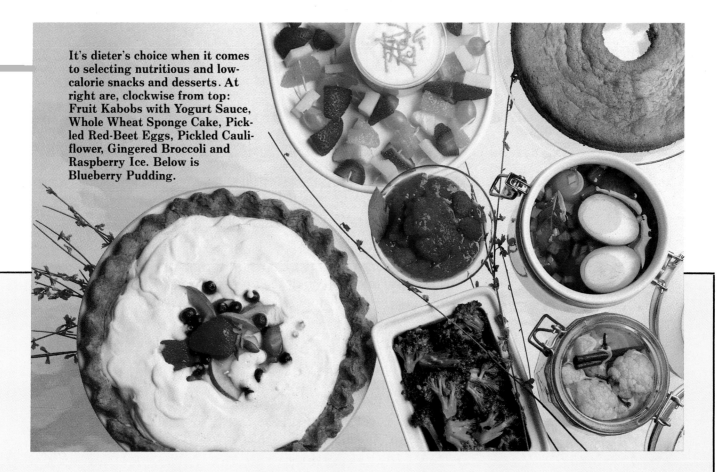

It's dieter's choice when it comes to selecting nutritious and low-calorie snacks and desserts. At right are, clockwise from top: Fruit Kabobs with Yogurt Sauce, Whole Wheat Sponge Cake, Pickled Red-Beet Eggs, Pickled Cauliflower, Gingered Broccoli and Raspberry Ice. Below is Blueberry Pudding.

Pineapple–Orange Delight

Makes 9 servings (121 calories each)

1 cup whole wheat graham cracker crumbs
3 tablespoons soft butter
⅓ cup nonfat dry milk
½ cup chilled orange juice
1 egg white
2 teaspoons lemon juice
2 tablespoons honey
1 can (8 ounces) unsweetened crushed pineapple, drained

Mix graham cracker crumbs and butter in a medium bowl until crumbly. Remove ⅓ cup of crumbs and set aside. Press the remaining crumbs in an ungreased 8 × 8-inch pan.

Beat the dry milk, orange juice and egg white on highest speed of electric mixer for about 3 minutes; add lemon juice and beat 3 minutes more. Slowly add honey and beat for another 30 seconds. Fold in the pineapple and pour into pan. Sprinkle with reserved crumbs. Freeze at least 8 hours.

Pickled Red-Beet Eggs

Makes 6 eggs (about 80 calories each)

6 medium eggs
1 cup cider vinegar
1 cup cooked red-beet liquid
2 tablespoons maple syrup or honey
1 medium onion, chopped
4 whole cloves
3 peppercorns
1 bay leaf

Hard-cook the eggs, peel them and place in a large bowl or 1-quart jar. Combine the remaining ingredients and pour the mixture over the eggs. Cover and refrigerate. (Although the eggs may not have completely changed color, they may be eaten after overnight refrigeration. The eggs will become purple after four days.)

Raspberry Ice

Makes 2 servings (77 calories each)

1½ cups raspberries
1 tablespoon honey, or to taste

Puree the raspberries and honey in a food processor. Strain and freeze. For smoother texture, process again and refreeze or serve immediately.

Gingered Broccoli

Makes 6 servings (about 60 calories each)

This dish can be served piping hot, but the flavor is really outstanding if it's allowed to marinate for a day after cooking. Serve cold as a low-calorie snack.

1 tablespoon vegetable oil
1 tablespoon minced peeled ginger root
3 shallots, minced
6 cups broccoli florets
½ cup chicken stock
2 teaspoons tamari or soy sauce
2 teaspoons rice vinegar
1 teaspoon cornstarch

Heat the oil in a large skillet or wok. Add the ginger and shallots and saute until the shallots have wilted. Add the broccoli and stir-fry for about a minute. In a medium bowl, combine the stock, tamari or soy sauce, vinegar and cornstarch, then pour over the broccoli. Cover and steam until the broccoli is crisp-tender. Serve immediately or refrigerate and serve chilled.

Beverages

Few things are more relaxing or satisfying than sharing a cool drink with friends on the front porch in summer, or curling up with a hot drink on a cold winter night. But such pleasures do not come without their share of calories. As a result, many people hate to "waste" calories on something that goes down so easily. They ignore everything but water, diet soft drinks and black coffee.

But beverages don't have to be a "waste" of calories. The Rodale Test Kitchen has developed a line of thirst-quenching drinks that can replace high-calorie alcoholic drinks and rich ice cream concoctions. Some of them—like the Carob-Peanut Shake—can occasionally substitute for a meal when you are in a rush. Try Cranberry Punch instead of gin at your next gathering. Replace your chemical-packed diet soft drinks with Cider Rose. You'll stay refreshed—and thin!

Carob-Peanut Shake

Makes 2 servings (141 calories each)

2 cups skim milk
1 tablespoon carob powder
2 tablespoons nonfat dry milk
1 tablespoon peanut butter
1 teaspoon vanilla
dash of ground cinnamon

Combine ingredients in a blender and whiz for 1 minute.

Spicy Sparkling Cider

Makes 4 servings (63 calories each)

2 red hibiscus tea bags
5 whole cloves
1 cinnamon stick, 2 inches long
1 very thin orange or lemon slice
2 cups boiling water
2 cups sparkling apple cider

Place the tea bags, cloves, cinnamon stick and orange or lemon slice in boiling water and steep for 15 minutes, or until the tea is richly red and aromatic. Strain and cool.

For each serving, pour ½ cup tea and ½ cup cider over crushed ice.

Mixed Fruit Sparkler

Makes 4 servings (35 calories each)

1 cup orange juice
1 cup sparkling mineral water or seltzer
2 tablespoons frozen apple juice concentrate
mint sprigs (garnish)

Combine ingredients in a small pitcher. Serve over ice, garnished with mint.

Cranberry Punch

Makes 4 servings (97 calories each)

½ cup cranberries
½ cup red raspberries or strawberries
1 banana
2 cups apple juice

Combine ingredients in a blender and whiz until smooth.

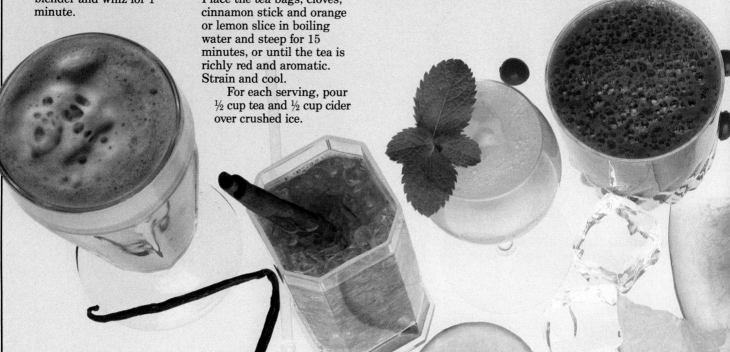

Calories at the Cocktail Hour

Most people have a preference for a certain type of drink when it comes to the cocktail hour, be it a martini, a bottle of beer or simply an innocent glass of club soda. If you wanted to limit yourself to spending 100 calories on drinking at your next party or gathering, what could you expect to get? The table below, which lists some of the more popular alcoholic beverages, will give you a clue.

Drink	Quantity	Calories	Serving Size per 100 Calories	Servings	Drink	Quantity	Calories	Serving Size per 100 Calories	Servings
Beer					Liqueurs & aperitifs				
Michelob	12 oz.	160	7.5 oz.	⅗ bottle	Black Russian	4 oz.	317	1.3 oz.	⅓ drink
Lite (Miller)	12 oz.	96	12.5 oz.	1 bottle	Dubonnet Red	3½ oz.	141	2.5 oz.	¾ drink
Natural Light (Anheuser-Busch)	12 oz.	110	10.9 oz.	9/10 bottle	Creme de menthe	⅔ oz.	67	1.0 oz.	1½ drinks
Mixed drinks					Wine				
Gin & tonic	8 oz.	265	3.0 oz.	⅓ drink	Red	3½ oz.	67	5.2 oz.	1½ drinks
Manhattan	3¼ oz.	233	1.4 oz.	⅖ drink	White	3½ oz.	80	4.4 oz.	1¼ drinks
Martini	2½ oz.	152	1.6 oz.	⅗ drink	White wine spritzer	5 oz.	69	7.3 oz.	1½ drinks
Scotch & soda	4½ oz.	118	3.8 oz.	⅘ drink					
Screwdriver	4 oz.	202	2.0 oz.	½ drink					

Watermelon Quencher

Makes 4 servings
(51 calories each)

4 cups chilled cubed
    watermelon
4 lemon slices (garnish)
4 orange slices (garnish)
    mint sprigs (garnish)

Place the watermelon in a blender and process until thoroughly blended and foamy. Pour into glasses and garnish with lemon and orange slices and mint.

Fruit Shake

Makes 8 servings
(114 calories each)

2 frozen bananas (about
    16 slices)
1 cup frozen strawberries
    (12 to 14 berries)
4 cups unsweetened
    pineapple juice
1 cup skim milk

Place one banana, ½ cup of strawberries, 2 cups juice and ½ cup milk in a blender and mix well. Pour mixture into another container, then blend the remaining ingredients.

Cider Rose

Makes 4 servings
(117 calories each)

2 cups (1 pint) fresh
    strawberries, halved
1½ cups sparkling apple
    cider
4 thin lime slices (garnish)

Puree the strawberries in a food processor or a blender. Combine the puree and the cider in a cocktail shaker. Serve over crushed ice. Garnish with lime slices.

Melon Nightcap

Makes 4 servings
(37 calories each)

1 camomile tea bag or
    1 teaspoon loose
    camomile
1 cup boiling water
¼ cantaloupe, cubed
¼ cup yogurt
½ cup pineapple juice

Steep tea bags or camomile in boiling water for 15 to 20 minutes, or until aroma is strong. Strain and cool. Pour the tea into a blender. Add the remaining ingredients and blend until smooth. Serve over crushed ice.

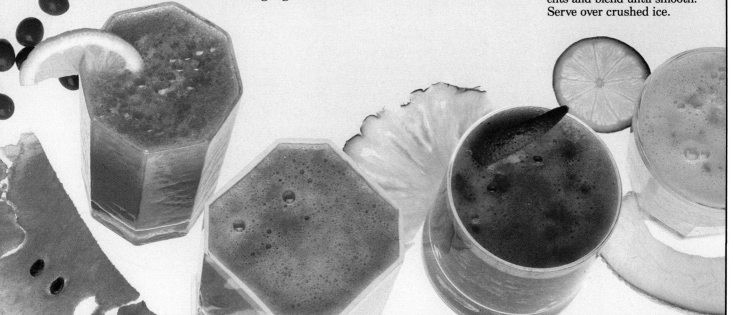

The 'Lite' Foods Revolution

Busy people. Single people. People with few culinary skills. Low-calorie food has long been a problem for them. But now there are slim-foods alternatives to high-calorie convenience foods and restaurant meals. Food manufacturers have responded to the need for quick, low-calorie products by marketing "lite foods" (the name is a streamlined, reduced version of the word light).

Lite foods run the gamut from reduced-sugar ketchup to low-calorie spaghetti. There are even whole lines of frozen dinners that can make a nice alternative to the days-of-old, fried-chicken-and-potatoes TV dinners that offered a lot of calories for a little volume.

But can lite foods help people lose weight? The answer, researchers are finding, is a resounding yes.

In a preliminary study by the Health, Weight and Stress Program at the Johns Hopkins Medical Institutions in Baltimore, researchers found that lite foods really did help people lose weight. The researchers worked with more than 100 overweight people and divided them into two groups. One group followed a standard, low-calorie reducing diet. The other group was asked to cut calories by eating lite foods. Over a 4-month period, the people who ate the lite foods each lost 5 to 7 pounds *more* than the people on the standard reducing diet.

According to one of the researchers, Maria Simonson, Ph.D., Sc.D., director of the program and coauthor of *The Complete University Medical Diet,* the dieters found the lite foods not only acceptable, but downright appealing. "The psychological effect was marvelous. These foods helped people maintain a nutritionally balanced, low-calorie diet without the usual feelings of boredom or deprivation. They stayed very motivated."

"If you feel better about a diet, you'll stick with it," says Janet Gailey-Phipps, Ph.D., another researcher on the study. "We actually found that people really liked the lite foods. After all, if you love certain foods, you have to be able to have them once in a while. Take desserts, for instance. People don't feel like giving them up forever. We found that the people in our study especially liked the lite desserts."

They found variety, too, to be very important. "The successful dieters in our study used a wide variety of lite food products, including fruit, cheese, margarine, bread, soup, and even beer," says Dr. Gailey-Phipps.

VARIETY IS THE SPICE OF LITE

Demand for full-course diet options has skyrocketed in the last few years. Two of the biggest competitors are Stouffer's Lean Cuisine and Weight Watchers' lite dinner line. One of the reasons for their great success is simply good taste—a taste that comes from the addition of flavorful light sauces and tasty herb mixtures.

Lean Cuisine, for instance, offers dishes such as Chicken and Vegetables with Vermicelli at only 260 calories a serving. Spaghetti with Beef and Mushroom Sauce has 280 calories. Fillet of Fish Florentine is a cod fillet rolled around spinach filling, cooked in a light sauce laced with sherry and topped with sesame bread crumbs. It seems impossible, but this dish has only 220 calories.

Weight Watchers offers a similar array of entrees (including pizza!) and a wide assortment of condiments and salad dressings, including mayonnaise at 40 calories per serving, blue cheese dressing at 20 calories per serving and brown gravy with mushrooms at 12 calories for a ¼-cup serving.

It is also possible to have an entire lite spaghetti dinner. First, there is lite pasta. Prince markets a few varieties. Farook Tausiq, vice president of quality control for Prince, says that the secret to their lite pasta is to "coat the regular pasta (made with enriched semolina flour) with a film of egg white. This coating allows the pasta to absorb more water without losing texture and flavor. Normally, 2 ounces of dry pasta cook up to 5 ounces. With Prince lite pasta, you only need 1.4 ounces dry to make 5 ounces cooked. That's a one-third reduction in calories."

You can top the lite pasta (Prince is only one of several brands on the market) with lite tomato sauce, like Ronzoni's Lite 'n' Natural sauce. Ronzoni's different lite sauces range from 45 to 50 calories per 4-ounce serving. That's a calorie saving of roughly 36 percent over the average sauce's calorie count of at least 80.

In addition to main courses, there are also lite versions of desserts and other treats. Jelly, for example, can be made with less sugar and more fruit. However, it may not be called jelly. According to James Weidman III, director of corporate communications for Welch's, "There's a standard of identity for jelly. If that's altered, then the name must be changed, too. We could have called it imitation jelly, but that has a negative sound to it, and it's not really imitation anyway. We simply reduced the sugar content by one-third and put more natural fruit in it." The product is called Welch's Lite Spread, and it comes in various flavors.

Canned fruit has also been slimmed down by many companies. There are several different methods of cutting down the calories in canned fruit without hurting the flavor. Del Monte's lite fruits are packed in a thin syrup or water that has been lightly sweetened with sugar or corn syrup.

Of course, convenience foods should be used only for the purpose for which they were intended—as a convenience when lack of time or availability makes having the real thing out of the question. After all, we all know it's just as easy to peel a banana as it is to open a can of fruit. But then again, it may not be fruit you're after. Maybe it's pizza you have a craving for. Or pasta. By selecting a Weight Watchers' frozen pizza you know that a single portion of 350 calories won't ruin your diet, and it's just enough to satisfy the craving. Better yet, there aren't any

extra pieces left in the box (like there are when you bring a pie home from the pizzeria) to tempt you into eating more.

The same goes for pasta. How often do you think of eating cannelloni on a diet? But with the Lean Cuisine dinner, you can treat yourself to the pasta, cheese and sauce dish for only 260 calories. That's just a crack in your daily calorie allotment. And again, there's no option for seconds.

Of course, if you're *really* hungry and planning on a frozen diet dish for dinner, portion size can mean a lot. Common sense tells you that Fillet of Fish Divan and Cheese Cannelloni with Tomato Sauce, both advertised at "less than 300 calories" can't be equal in size. And they aren't. The fish dish gives you 12⅜ ounces. The cannelloni gives you 9⅛ ounces. The pizza we mentioned is only 6 ounces.

A LITTLE LITE READING

Which brings us to a caveat in lite-food eating. Read labels. If bulk is important to you, you'll want to check portion size. Federal regulation says that in order for a food to be labeled low calorie, it can have no more than 40 calories per serving. "Reduced calorie" means that the food is at least one-third lower in calories than the regular kind.

Also, and most important, if it's weight loss you're after, "lite" or "light" doesn't always mean fewer calories. Manufacturers use the words to indicate reductions in other things such as salt, sugar or cholesterol. So, dieter beware. Read the labels carefully.

The trick to using lite foods is to use them as you would any other dish. That means relax and enjoy your meal, keep track of what you eat and don't overeat. Lite foods can be a tasty, healthy and convenient answer to your slim-foods needs on those days when time is *not* on your side. You might want to keep a small supply on hand for such an "emergency." That way, you'll never have an excuse not to eat light.

3

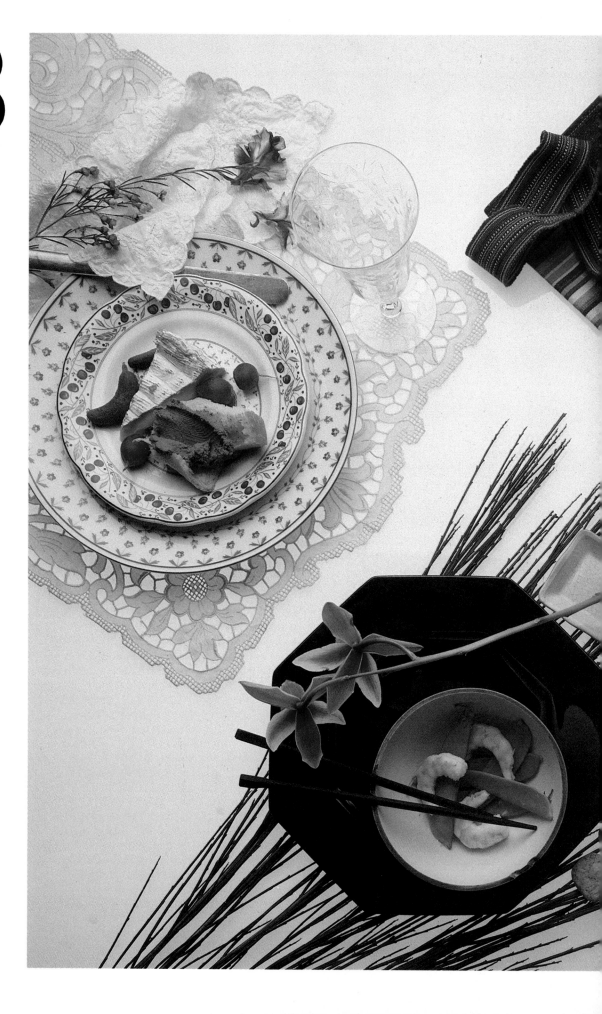

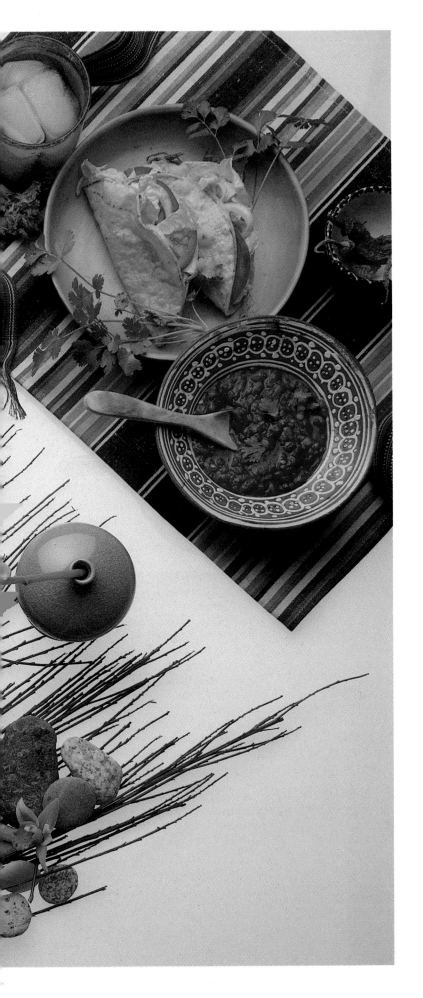

Indulge Your Ethnic Heritage

Your favorite ethnic foods don't have to be your undoing. In fact, experts advise against giving them up.

In 1908, when New York City public schools began serving lunches, officials made sure that children in the Italian section could eat macaroni and two slices of Italian bread while kids in the Irish section got cheese sandwiches and cocoa. Children of other ethnic backgrounds also received the types of food they encountered at home—foods that they not only were used to, but liked as well.

In most cases, foods that people are used to *are* the ones they like the best. "While there is little evidence that differences in food preference are genetically programmed," says Paul Rozin, Ph.D., a psychologist at the University of Pennsylvania, "it is clear that after food patterns have been established, those foods are the ones that tend to be satisfying. Immigrants to America eat many kinds of foods, but they continue a strong preference for native foods."

In researching her book *Ethnic Cuisine: The Flavor Principle Cookbook,* Dr. Rozin's wife, Elizabeth, found that "many Americans with a strong ethnic heritage—and we're talking about a lot of people—do eat American fare on a daily basis. But once or twice or three times a week they also sit down to a meal of 'real food'—ethnic cuisine. For them, not only is the taste important, but there's a great deal of social satisfaction involved, too."

It's no wonder that when people go on a diet they say they can't live without their spaghetti, or their pierogi, or whatever their favorite food "just happens" to be! Nor should they be expected to. "Asking overweight people to give up their ethnic foods is asking a great deal—and it is not desirable psychologically," says Dr. Rozin. "Some ethnic foods are high in calories, yes. But which would you get more satisfaction from, a bowl of skim milk or a scoop of ice cream? The same goes for ethnic foods. But a high-calorie dish in itself isn't fattening—it's eating too much of it that is. The good thing about ethnic food is you *can* eat less of a high-satiety food and get more satisfaction out of it in the end."

A LESSON FROM "THE OLD COUNTRY"

Mrs. Rozin feels we should take an interest not only in *what* people from other lands eat but also in the *way* they eat it. She says we should try to recapture the way food is served back in "the old country"— wherever that may be. If you were to compare your ethnic-American table with a table from the Homeland, she says, chances are you'd find some important differences.

An American who travels overseas to visit relatives in Czechoslovakia during the summer, for instance, would enjoy garden-fresh vegetables like tomatoes, green peppers, string beans and potatoes at every single meal. Sure, Czechs eat kielbasa— their version of sausage—but they eat it *with* vegetables. Juicy ripe apricots, plums, currants and gooseberries might accompany the meal. The Slovak-American family back home may be content just to dig into the kielbasa or, perhaps, may compromise the fresh food with frozen vegetables, dried apricots or canned sauerkraut. As a result, they're likely to eat more of the fat-filled kielbasa and less of the leaner accompaniments than their relatives across the sea. Also, the American table is likely to hold several nontraditional foods—foods that are American in style. Generally speaking, the American table holds *more* of *all* foods.

So, where your weight is concerned, getting back to the way Grandma made it—and served it—isn't a bad idea at all. "For the most part," Mrs. Rozin says,

"traditional recipes don't present a problem in terms of overweight— partly because different cultures have different, more tolerant attitudes toward overweight (plump women are considered desirable in some countries, such as Turkey) —but mostly because there's not an abundance of food available to start with.

"Here, in America, we have so much food that we overdo it," she says. "The way we eat meat is a good example. Many ethnic traditions rely far less on animal products than we do; they rely more on plant foods. The Chinese, for example, will usually cut up meat and distribute it throughout the dish. When other cuisines use dairy foods and meats, a little bit goes a long way."

MEAT-EATING NATIONS ARE HEAVIER

So, what does a love for meat mean in terms of overweight? Well, when we look at international food statistics, it's clear that the more animal protein people eat, the heavier they are. In Asia, where overweight generally is not a problem, the average person eats four times more protein from plant sources than from animal sources. In the USSR, where people are considerably heftier, the ratio of plant to animal protein is nearly 50-50. And in the United States, where two out of five people are overweight, the average person eats over twice as much animal protein as plant protein.

Scientists agree that eating meat is not in itself the *cause* of obesity. However, the more meat you eat, the more fat you are getting in your diet. And, not surprisingly, studies show obesity is more of a problem in countries where the diet contains a high percentage of total calories from fat.

CARBOHYDRATES SATISFY

So, if high fat intake can make a nation as a whole fat, what's the magic food that keeps some nations as a whole trim? The answer is

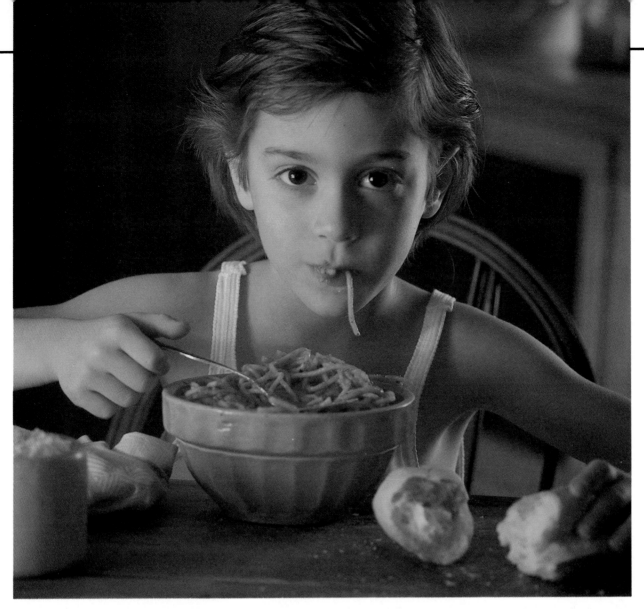

complex—complex carbohydrates, that is. Almost across the board, people whose total diet includes a high percentage of complex carbohydrates—grains, beans, rice, pasta and so forth—suffer less obesity and fewer obesity-related diseases. One thing that makes complex carbohydrates so attractive as slim foods is the fact that they are rich in fiber. When you eat them, "a sense of satiety is achieved before excessive energy [in the form of calories] is consumed," explains Denis Burkitt, M.D., a leading expert on fiber. With foods low in fiber, it's easy to take in too many calories before you feel satisfied and "this fosters the development of obesity," he says.

And that's what makes most ethnic cuisines so inviting. Many are low in meat, making a little go a long way, and are brimming with the fresh vegetables, wholesome grains and fragrant herbs and spices that are part of each nation's culinary heritage. And while many are laden with oils, creams and noodles, you can learn to prepare your favorite dishes in a way that won't put on extra pounds. They may not be *made* the way Grandma made them, but they can *taste* that way.

To prove the point—and to pique your ethnic taste buds again (this time without the guilt)—the Rodale Test Kitchen has taken the world's most popular cuisines and developed recipes that are lower in calories, yet totally traditional in nature and flavor. Some of the cuisines presented, such as Mexican and Japanese, are naturally low in calories, so you'll have little to learn in cutting back on calories. With others, such as French and German, you'll find calorie-saving tips you can apply to some of your other favorite dishes.

Give up spaghetti? No way! Our fondness for certain foods usually begins when we are young, and family tradition and ethnic custom have a lot to do with what those foods will be. Psychologists feel it is foolhardy to attempt to give up our favorite foods for the sake of a reducing diet. Such diets are only setups for failure. Rather, we should learn to eat such foods in moderation.

Italy

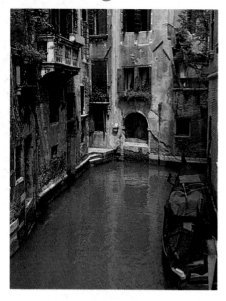

Italian food has become so popular in the U.S. that today it's nothing short of Big Business. Spaghetti sauce sales are swelling, and companies with such un-Italian-sounding names as Borden, Pillsbury and Hershey are jockeying for position in the great macaroni market.

Of course, there's more to Italian fare than pasta and tomato sauce. Polenta, gnocchi, bean dishes, sausage, fish chowders and antipasto are all Italian favorites. But the best-known Italian-American foods are spaghetti, lasagna, ravioli and pizza.

Part of the reason pasta sells so well (aside from its satisfying taste and texture) is an increasing public awareness of the importance of complex carbohydrates in the diet. At long last, pasta is shedding its image as a fattening, nonnutritious food and taking its rightful place as a health-promoting food.

Back "on the Continent," Italy still ranks high in intake of cereals—especially wheat, because of pasta—and ranks low in meat consumption compared to West Germany, France, the Netherlands, Belgium and Luxembourg, as well as Ireland and the United Kingdom. Italians also take in less fat than people in those countries, despite the fact that total fat intake per person has nearly doubled in the last 20 years. Because of this, Italian nutritionist Flaminio Fidanzo is attempting to get his countrymen to cut down on fat consumption. With this spirit in mind, we offer this low-fat version of Italian cuisine.

Pizza with Zucchini Crust

Makes 1 12-inch pizza (362 calories per ¼ pie)

Crust
4 cups grated zucchini
4 eggs
½ cup whole wheat pastry flour
1 teaspoon dried basil

Sauce
1 medium onion, finely chopped
2 cloves garlic, minced
1 medium green pepper, seeded and coarsely chopped
1 can (16 ounces) whole tomatoes, with juice, coarsely chopped

Topping
8 ounces part-skim mozzarella cheese, shredded
2 cloves garlic, minced
¼ cup chopped fresh flatleaf parsley
1 teaspoon dried thyme
¼ cup freshly grated Parmesan cheese
1½ tablespoons minced fresh chives (garnish)

To prepare the crust, remove as much water from the zucchini as possible by placing a handful inside a cotton kitchen towel and wringing it. Place in a large bowl. Repeat until all the zucchini is free of moisture. (There should be about 2 cups after wringing.)

Beat the eggs in a small bowl and add to zucchini. Add the flour and basil and mix thoroughly. Spread in the bottom of a 12-inch pizza pan and bake in a preheated 375°F oven for 20 minutes, or until well browned.

To prepare the sauce, place the onions, garlic, peppers and tomatoes and juice in a small saucepan. Bring to a boil, then reduce heat and simmer for 25 minutes, or until excess liquid has been absorbed. Puree the sauce in a food processor until smooth.

To prepare the topping, toss the mozzarella with the garlic, parsley and thyme.

Remove crust from oven and allow to cool slightly. Sprinkle Parmesan over crust, then spread with tomato sauce. Sprinkle the mozzarella mixture over top. Bake at 375°F for 20 minutes, until cheese is melted and lightly browned. Remove from oven, sprinkle with chives and serve.

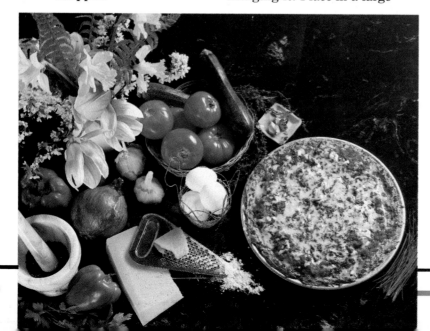

Shrimp Fra Diablo

Makes 6 servings (235 calories each)

This spicy dish is naturally low in calories. For a milder sauce, omit the Tabasco and/or remove the peppers after the sauce simmers.

2 tablespoons olive oil
¼ cup minced onion
4 cloves garlic, crushed
2 hot chili peppers, split and seeded
½ cup tomato paste
½ cup lemon juice
½ cup red wine vinegar
1 cup water
1 tablespoon tamari or soy sauce
dash of Tabasco sauce
pinch of cayenne pepper
1½ tablespoons minced fresh basil
1¾ pounds shrimp, shelled and cleaned

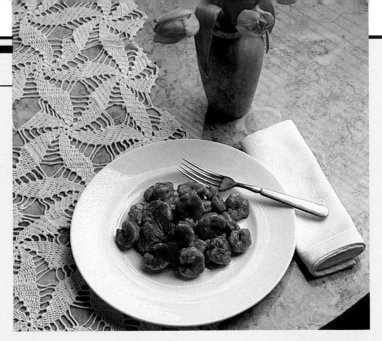

Heat the oil in a large skillet. Add the onions, garlic and peppers and saute for 5 minutes. Add the tomato paste, lemon juice, vinegar, water, tamari or soy sauce, Tabasco and cayenne. Simmer, uncovered, for 10 minutes. Let cool to room temperature. Stir in the basil.

Marinate the shrimp in the sauce for 30 minutes. Place the shrimp on a broiler pan, about 4 inches away from heat. Broil 4 to 5 minutes on each side, basting often with the sauce.

Top with remaining sauce and serve or serve sauce as an accompaniment.

Chicken Cacciatore

Makes 6 servings (387 calories each)

Traditionally, this dish calls for sauteing the chicken in copious amounts of olive oil. This version eliminates that step. Instead it calls for broiling the chicken to brown it, significantly reducing the calories.

1 chicken (broiler-fryer, 4 to 5 pounds), skinned and cut into serving pieces
2 tablespoons corn oil
1 large green pepper, chopped
1 large onion, chopped
½ cup chopped celery
3 cloves garlic, minced
1 cup sliced mushrooms
6 large tomatoes, peeled, seeded and coarsely chopped, or 2 cups canned tomatoes, coarsely chopped
1 bay leaf
2 tablespoons chopped parsley
1 cup chicken stock

1 teaspoon dried basil
¼ teaspoon dried thyme
¼ teaspoon crushed hot red peppers (optional)

Place chicken in a hot broiler and broil until all sides are golden. Set chicken aside.

Heat the oil in a large skillet, add the green peppers, onions, celery and garlic and saute until the vegetables are soft but not browned. Add the mushrooms and saute for 2 minutes. Add the tomatoes, bay leaf, parsley, stock, basil, thyme, and red peppers (if used). Bring to a boil, then reduce heat and simmer for 10 minutes.

Add the chicken to the sauce, cover and simmer gently for 30 minutes, or until the chicken is tender. Remove cover during last 10 minutes to thicken sauce. Skim off excess fat. Remove bay leaf before serving.

Pesto

Makes about ¾ cup (123 calories per tablespoon)

Pesto is a Genoese basil sauce made with a butter and olive oil base. To cut calories, we have omitted the butter. If a low-calorie dish is what you're after, you'd do best to serve this sauce over spaghetti squash, *not* pasta.

2 cups fresh basil
3 tablespoons walnuts
2 cloves garlic, peeled
½ cup olive oil
½ cup freshly grated Parmesan cheese

Place all ingredients except the Parmesan in a food processor fitted with the steel blade. Process, stopping from time to time to scrape the sides. Fold in the cheese and mix by hand.

When saucing pasta, mix 2 tablespoons of hot water with the pesto, then toss with the hot pasta.

France

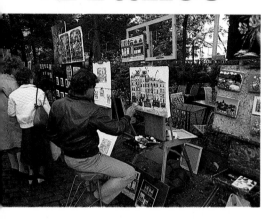

We go to *restaurants,* order *entrees,* compliment the *chef,* serve *hors d'oeuvres* at parties, enjoy pie *a la mode,* join *gourmet* clubs and talk about which *cuisine* we like the best. If it seems like our language of *gastronomy* has a decidedly French flavor, it's a direct tribute to France and her influence in elevating the preparation of food to a form of art.

While Frenchmen eat foods similar to those eaten by other western Europeans, their cuisine is lighter and more delicate. Where the English favor a well-roasted side of beef, the French may braise it first, sprinkle it with capers, encase it in a lighter-than-air puff pastry and bake it until tender.

Butter is a characteristic French flavoring, along with cream, wine, chicken or meat stock, cheese, herbs and mustard. Interestingly, foods that are high in fat—such as duck, pork and lamb—are usually prepared with wine or fruit (as in duck a l'orange), while low-fat foods wind up in the cream and butter sauces. The French also usually eat their bread plain—never smeared with butter. And they eat much more fish and poultry than red meats. As a whole, the French are not snackers. Perhaps this contributes to the fact that the French as a people are not particularly known for their obesity; they're more likely to complain about their livers.

Chicken Terrine with Tarragon and Lemon

Makes 10 servings (187 calories each)

1 chicken (broiler-fryer, 3 to 4
    pounds), cut up
1 cup chopped onions
½ cup chopped carrots
½ cup chopped celery
3 small lemons, thinly sliced
2 teaspoons dried tarragon
   bouquet garni (bay leaf, few
     sprigs of dried thyme,
     parsley sprig, 1 clove,
     6 peppercorns, tied in a
     piece of cheesecloth)
¼ teaspoon pepper
5 cups water
½ pound zucchini, cut into
    large strips
2 tablespoons unflavored gelatin

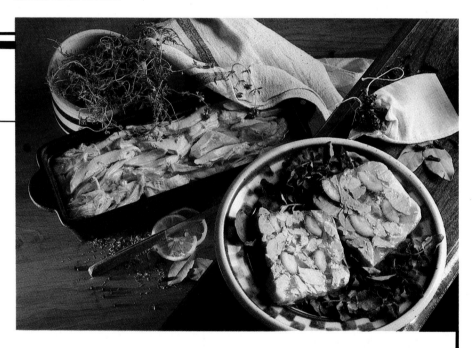

Wash the chicken, then place it in a large pot along with the onions, carrots, celery, lemon slices, tarragon, bouquet garni, pepper and water. Bring the liquid to a boil, then immediately reduce heat. Allow the chicken to cook over very low heat for 1 to 1½ hours, until the meat begins to fall from the bones. Remove the chicken from the pot, drain and allow to cool. Strain and reserve the stock.

Steam the zucchini strips briefly, just until crisp-tender. Remove immediately and plunge into cold water to stop the cooking process. Blot excess water from zucchini and set aside.

Bone the chicken, discarding skin and bones. (The chicken should remain in large pieces.) Place one layer of chicken in a 4½ × 8½-inch loaf pan. Arrange a layer of zucchini slices on top, then another layer of chicken, then a layer of zucchini and finally a layer of chicken.

Strain 3½ cups of the reserved stock into a small pot. Bring to a boil and dissolve the gelatin in the stock. Pour into the pan, then tap the pan several times on the counter to make sure liquid is well distributed. Pour any extra gelatin mixture into a shallow glass container. Cover the terrine with foil and chill it and the gelatin in the refrigerator overnight. Unmold the terrine on a serving platter, then break the chilled gelatin into cubes and place them around the mold as a garnish.

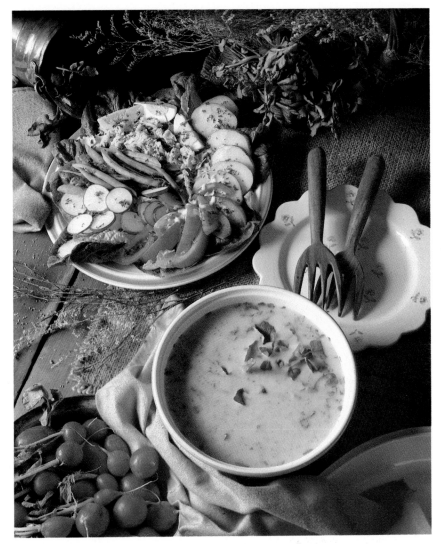

"Cream" of Watercress Soup and Salad Nicoise

Salad Nicoise

Makes 4 servings (341 calories each)

Calories in salad Nicoise can be cut by using water-packed instead of oil-packed tuna and serving it with the buttermilk vinaigrette suggested here. This dressing uses no oil.

1 head romaine lettuce,
        separated into leaves
1 pound fresh green beans
4 hard-cooked eggs, quartered
4 new potatoes, boiled and
        thinly sliced
1 can (6½ to 7 ounces) water-
        packed tuna, drained, or
        ½ pound fresh tuna,
        lightly poached
4 ripe tomatoes, cut into wedges
8 red radishes, sliced
¼ cup chopped parsley
    Buttermilk Vinaigrette

Wash the romaine and separate the leaves into four portions.
    Clean and string the green beans. Steam until crisp-tender. Remove from heat, drain at once and plunge into cold water to stop the cooking process.
    Arrange the lettuce on four large plates. Arrange one-fourth of the green beans on top, then the eggs, potatoes and tuna. Top with tomato wedges and radish slices and sprinkle with parsley. Serve with buttermilk vinaigrette.

BUTTERMILK VINAIGRETTE

1 tablespoon Dijon mustard
2 scallions, white only, chopped
¼ teaspoon dried tarragon
1 cup buttermilk
    white pepper, to taste

Whisk all ingredients together in a medium bowl. Taste and adjust seasoning. Allow to stand at room temperature for 1 hour before serving so flavors blend. (This recipe makes about 1 cup, with 8 calories per tablespoon.)

"Cream" of Watercress Soup

Makes 6 servings (about 100 calories each)

Traditionally prepared, this soup uses cream for enrichment, texture and body. This low-calorie version is thickened with potatoes instead. The soup is a lovely shade of green, the result of stirring the chopped leaves into the heated soup and serving immediately.

2 bunches watercress (use fresh
        cress only, with shiny
        leaves and crisp stems)
3 small potatoes, cut into ¼-inch
        slices
1 leek, white only, thinly sliced
5 cups water or light chicken
        broth

Separate the watercress leaves from the stems. Coarsely chop the stems and place them in a large pot along with the potatoes, leeks and water. Bring to a boil, then simmer until the potatoes are very soft, about 45 minutes.
    Meanwhile, finely chop the watercress leaves. When the potatoes have softened, puree the soup in a food processor or blender. Return the puree to the pot, thinning, if necessary, with additional broth, water or skim milk. Turn the heat up and bring to a boil. Remove from heat, stir in the chopped leaves, taste and adjust seasoning and serve.

Provencal-Style Fish Soup with Rouille

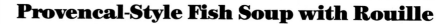

Makes 6 servings (187 calories each)

This flavorful soup, like many Mediterranean dishes, is inherently low in calories; the only alteration it requires is the elimination of olive oil, an essential ingredient in a traditional version. The soup is commonly strained before serving; if you choose to serve it this way, the result is a rather thin broth. You can choose to serve the soup right from the pot, without straining, since the texture is more interesting.

½ cup finely chopped leeks
½ cup finely chopped onions
¼ cup finely chopped carrots
   5 cloves garlic, minced
   1 pound tomatoes, peeled, seeded and chopped
   1 teaspoon dried thyme
3 tablespoons chopped parsley
5 cups water, fish stock or light chicken stock
2 pounds mixed, nonoily fish or, if the soup will be strained, 3 pounds fish heads, skeletons and scraps, washed
black pepper, to taste
Rouille

Place the leeks, onions, carrots, garlic, tomatoes, thyme, parsley, water and fish in a large pot. Bring to a boil and reduce heat immediately. Simmer for 45 minutes, or until the fish flakes easily.

To strain, pour the soup through a fine-mesh sieve, pressing on the solids to extract as much juice as possible. Discard the solids when they are squeezed dry. If you plan to serve the soup unstrained, remove the fish with a slotted spoon, chop into small pieces and return to the pot.

Taste and adjust seasoning. Reheat. Serve in warmed soup plates and allow each person to stir in rouille to taste.

ROUILLE

1 medium red bell pepper, finely chopped
1 medium potato, boiled and coarsely chopped
3 large cloves garlic, peeled
½ teaspoon Tabasco sauce
2 tablespoons low-calorie mayonnaise

Simmer the peppers in water to cover for 5 minutes. Drain, reserving cooking liquid. Place the peppers, potatoes, garlic, Tabasco and mayonnaise in a blender or food processor and puree. The mixture should be the consistency of thick mayonnaise; thin with pepper cooking water, if necessary. For a spicier flavor, add additional garlic or Tabasco. (This recipe makes 1 cup, with 9 calories per tablespoon.)

Salmon with Lemon-Dill Sabayon, below left, and Provencal Style Fish Soup with Rouille, below right.

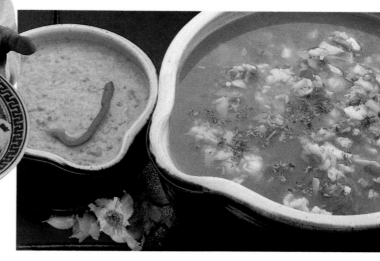

Stuffed Chicken Florentine

Makes 4 servings (236 calories each)

1¼ pounds boned skinned chicken breast (about 2 medium breasts), cut into 4 halves
½ cup chopped scallions
2 cloves garlic, minced
¾ cup chicken stock
¾ cup chopped, lightly steamed spinach
¼ cup low-fat ricotta cheese
3 tablespoons Parmesan cheese
¼ teaspoon dried tarragon
⅛ teaspoon black pepper
¼ teaspoon dried thyme
2 cups mushroom caps, halved
2 tablespoons chopped parsley
2 teaspoons lemon juice

Flatten the chicken breasts with a meat mallet. (Do not pound too thin or chicken will tear.)

In a small skillet, saute the scallions and garlic in 3 tablespoons of stock for 3 minutes. Remove from heat and stir in the spinach, cheeses, tarragon, pepper and thyme. Place ¼ cup of spinach mixture on each chicken breast and roll up lengthwise. Secure with string.

Spray a 10-inch skillet with vegetable coating. Saute rolled chicken breasts until lightly browned on all sides, about 10 minutes. Place chicken in an 8-inch square baking dish.

Pour remaining chicken stock into skillet used for browning the chicken. To deglaze the pan, stir quickly while scraping the bottom of the pan to dissolve all the brown bits. Pour over the chicken.

Spread mushrooms and parsley over chicken. Bake, covered, in a preheated 350°F oven for 20 minutes. Uncover, baste and bake an additional 20 minutes, until filling is very hot and chicken is cooked. Sprinkle lemon juice over chicken and baste again. Remove string and serve.

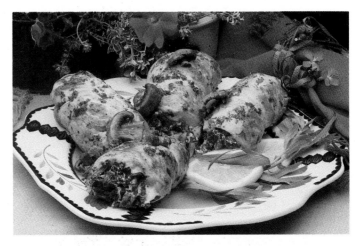

Stuffed Chicken Florentine

Salmon with Lemon-Dill Sabayon

Makes 6 servings (170 calories each)

Sabayons are generally sweet sauces that are served with desserts. This savory version uses the ingredients of the traditional hollandaise—lemon and dill—that is commonly paired with salmon, but cuts the calories and fat considerably.

2 egg yolks
1 tablespoon fresh lemon juice
⅓ cup chicken stock
2 tablespoons butter
3 teaspoons chopped fresh dill
1½ pounds salmon fillets
⅛ teaspoon freshly ground white pepper

Have the sauce ingredients at room temperature. Whisk the egg yolks and lemon juice in the top of a double boiler over simmering water until thick. Slowly whisk in the stock and continue whisking until the sauce becomes even thicker. (Do not allow it to get too hot or it will curdle.) Remove from heat and whisk in butter and dill.

Meanwhile, broil the salmon. (The broiling time will vary depending upon the thickness of the fish. It is best to test the fish for doneness while broiling.)

Add the pepper to the sauce, taste and adjust seasoning. Top the fish with some of the sauce. Serve at once.
NOTE: The sauce, which takes about 10 minutes to prepare, is best served soon after making it. Do not reheat or it will curdle.

Steak au Poivre

Makes 4 servings (315 calories each)

4 filet mignons, strip sirloins or club steaks (6 ounces each), 1 inch thick
2 tablespoons coarsely crushed peppercorns, or more, to taste
1 lemon, quartered

Have the steaks at room temperature. Scatter half the crushed peppercorns on a cutting board in an area about the size of steaks. Lay the steaks on top of the pepper and press them firmly into the pepper with the heel of your hand. Scatter the rest of the pepper on the cutting board and repeat with other side of steaks.

Heat a heavy skillet over medium-high heat until it is quite hot—the meat should sizzle when it touches the pan. Add enough peanut oil to lightly coat the bottom of the pan, then add the steaks. Sear for 2 minutes on each side, reduce heat to medium and cook to the desired degree of doneness. Squeeze one lemon quarter over each steak before serving.

Germany

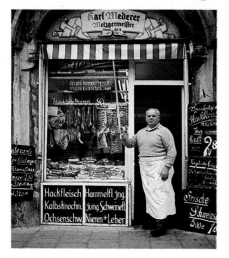

The German government has a lot of weighty issues to consider these days, but there is one that truly takes the cake (the Black Forest cherry cake, that is). Too many Germans are too fat, officials say, and it's taking a toll on the nation's health. They point to these major ways to knock pounds off: Cut back on fats, calories and alcohol, and eat more vegetables.

If their diet is getting the Germans into trouble, it's not because there's anything inherently nonnutritious about cabbage, corn, apples, pork, noodles and whole grain breads—all foods the Germans are fond of. But German cooks have a heavy hand with butter and other fats and sugar. Noodles are drenched in meaty gravies. Dumplings float in soups. And no main meal is complete without a hefty portion of meat.

When Germans settled in the United States, they "maintained their old-country cookery almost intact," says James Trager in *The Foodbook*. Wherever there were Germans, he says, there were dishes like *sauerbraten* (beef pot roast marinated in vinegar, seasonings and sugar), varieties of *wurst* (sausage), potato dumplings, *sauerkraut*, pretzels and *schnecken* (coffee cake).

Because of their love for these fattier foods, there is no such thing as "light German cuisine"—not yet, anyway. So how can you have your *kuchen* and eat it, too? Start by trying the fat-trimmed dishes we offer here.

Lamb with Mustard Sauce

Makes 4 servings (about 252 calories each)

8 small or 4 large loin lamb chops
1 tablespoon corn oil
¼ cup strong chicken stock
2 large shallots, minced
1 clove garlic, minced
¼ cup Pommery or Dijon mustard
1 tablespoon minced fresh parsley
black pepper, to taste

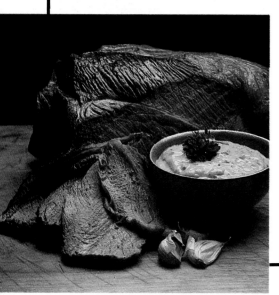

Heat a cast-iron skillet large enough to hold all the lamb chops. Add the oil, spreading it evenly over the bottom of the skillet. When the skillet is hot, add the chops and sear until well browned, about 1 minute on each side.

Place the pan in a hot broiler and broil the chops to desired doneness (the exact time will vary depending on the thickness of the chops). Remove chops to a heated plate and keep warm. Pour off excess fat and return skillet to high heat.

Add the stock, shallots and garlic to the pan and saute, stirring to prevent sticking. When the vegetables are well wilted (about 2 minutes), add the mustard and stir to mix well. When it is hot, stir in the parsley. Taste, and add pepper to taste. Place the lamb chops on individual heated plates, top each with a portion of the sauce and serve.
NOTE: The sauce is quite strong, so the lamb should not be sauced too heavily.

Wiener Schnitzel

Makes 6 servings (369 calories each)

By pan frying the cutlets in oil, instead of slowly simmering in butter, much less fat is absorbed.

1½ pounds veal cutlets, ½ inch thick
¾ cup whole wheat pastry flour
¼ teaspoon white pepper
2 tablespoons Parmesan cheese
2 eggs
2 tablespoons water
2 tablespoons peanut oil
4 lemon slices (garnish)

Pound veal cutlets with the edge of a plate or a heavy mallet until ¼ inch thick. Mix the flour, pepper and cheese in a small bowl. Beat the eggs with the water in a small bowl.

Lightly flour the cutlets by dipping each in the egg, then in flour, shaking off excess flour.

Heat 2 tablespoons oil in a heavy skillet. Quickly saute' cutlets, turning once. Keep warm until all cutlets are sauteed. Serve, garnished with lemon slices.

Duck with Apple Stuffing

Makes 4 servings (575 calories each)

Removing the skin and fat from the duck before cooking cuts back considerably on the calories in this dish. The duck, however, stays moist by the method of wrapping, basting and glazing used here.

 1 duck (4½ to 5 pounds)
 ¼ cup chopped onion
 ¼ cup chopped celery
 1 tablespoon butter
 1 tablespoon chopped parsley
 ½ teaspoon tamari or soy sauce
 ⅛ teaspoon pepper
1½ cups whole wheat bread
      cubes
 2 cups diced apples
 ½ cup diced zucchini
 ¼ cup raisins
 ⅓ cup orange juice
   Apple Glaze

Remove the giblets from the duck and set aside. Remove the skin and fat from the duck and discard; set duck aside.

Place the onions, celery and butter in a skillet and saute over medium heat until onions are translucent. Remove from heat and stir in parsley, tamari or soy sauce and pepper.

In a medium bowl, toss together the bread cubes, apples, zucchini and raisins. Add the onion mixture and mix. Add the orange juice and mix gently.

Stuff the prepared duck; do not pack. Wrap duck in muslin and tie securely with string.

Place duck breast side up in a roasting pan with 1 cup water and the giblets. Cover and roast in a preheated 350°F oven for 2 hours, or until done. Baste frequently with pan juices to keep muslin moist.

Remove muslin from duck and place on a heatproof serving platter. Brush with apple glaze and return to oven for 15 to 20 minutes. Serve with remaining apple glaze.

APPLE GLAZE

2 cups apple juice
1 teaspoon grated orange rind
1 teaspoon white wine vinegar
1 tablespoon honey
2 tablespoons water
1 tablespoon cornstarch

Place the apple juice, orange rind, vinegar and honey in a small saucepan over medium-high heat and cook until volume is reduced by half, about 45 minutes. Mix the water and cornstarch and gradually pour into hot juice, stirring constantly. Cook until thickened. (This recipe makes 1 cup, with 18 calories per tablespoon.)

Sweet-and-Sour Red Cabbage and Apple

Makes 4 servings (95 calories each)

Calories are saved in this dish by sauteing in water instead of butter or lard as is done in traditional versions.

3 cups thinly sliced red cabbage
1 onion, coarsely chopped
¼ cup water
2 apples (preferably McIntosh),
      peeled, seeded
      and thinly
      sliced

¼ cup red wine vinegar
 2 tablespoons honey
¼ teaspoon cloves

Place the cabbage and onions in a heavy skillet with the water and saute for 5 minutes over medium-high heat. Add the apples and saute for 2 to 3 minutes. Reduce heat, add the vinegar, honey and cloves and braise for 5 minutes, shaking the pan occasionally so the mixture doesn't stick. Taste, adjust

seasoning and serve as an accompaniment to hearty meat dishes.

Duck with Apple Stuffing,
Wiener Schnitzel and
Sweet-and-Sour
Red Cabbage and Apple

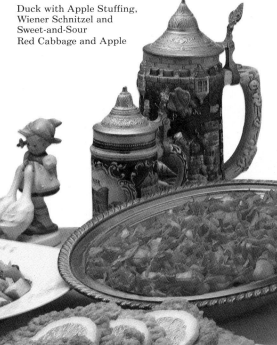

Mexico

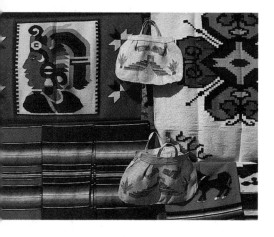

Jesse James refused to hold up the bank in McKinney, Texas. Why? It was the home of the bandit's favorite chili parlor! (Or so the legend goes.)

It was a sign of things to come. It wasn't so long ago that Mexican food was confined to the Southwest. Now, as far north as Barrow, Alaska, Eskimos can walk into a Mexican restaurant, doff their parkas and dig into a south-of-the-border meal of enchiladas and refried beans (a change from the usual caribou in seal oil).

Mexican cuisine is straightforward fare, based on beans (mostly pinto), some meat (chicken, beef or pork) and cornmeal *tortillas,* flat bread that can be fried to make *tacos,* or stuffed with fillings and folded to make *enchiladas,* or steamed to make *tamales.*

While all-day snacking is a custom in the Mexican villages, says University of Maryland anthropologist Aubrey W. Williams, Ph.D., snacks tend to be more along the line of berries and fruit, and may serve to bolster people's blood sugar levels.

Mexicans are also very active. They do "far less sitting around than we do, and walk just about everywhere they have to go," says Dr. Williams. "Obesity is not a problem."

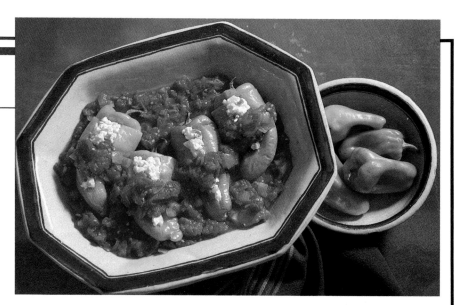

Skinny Chiles Rellenos

Makes 6 servings (232 calories each)

12 frying peppers
4 tablespoons vegetable stock or chicken stock
½ cup chopped onion
2 cloves garlic, minced
1 to 2 jalapeno peppers (fresh or canned), chopped
1⅓ cups corn kernels
1½ cups dry small-curd cottage cheese
½ cup shredded part-skim mozzarella cheese
⅛ to ¼ teaspoon freshly ground black pepper
⅛ teaspoon cayenne pepper
¼ teaspoon ground cumin
Mexican Tomato Sauce

The peppers either can be roasted and peeled or precooked by blanching. To roast, char peppers over a gas flame until the skin blisters and blackens. Place peppers between damp towels or in a brown paper bag for 30 minutes. The skin should slip off fairly easily when peppers are rinsed under cool tap water. To blanch, steam the peppers over boiling water until tender, about 6 minutes. Set peppers aside.

In a large skillet, heat the stock and saute the onions, garlic and jalapenos until onions wilt, about 2 minutes. Add the corn and cook until tender, about 8 minutes. Allow to cool slightly.

In a medium bowl, stir together the cottage cheese and mozzarella, black pepper, cayenne and cumin. Add corn mixture and mix well.

Make a T-shaped slit in each pepper, remove seeds and place enough of the mixture into each pepper to fill it, yet allow it to close easily.

Place 1 cup of Mexican tomato sauce in a 9 × 13-inch pan. Lay the peppers in the pan slit-side up and pour remaining sauce over peppers. Bake in a preheated 350°F oven until peppers are bubbly, about 20 minutes.

MEXICAN TOMATO SAUCE

1 onion, coarsely chopped
2 cloves garlic, minced
2 to 3 jalapeno peppers (fresh or canned), chopped
2 cups canned tomatoes, with juice, chopped

Place the onions, garlic, peppers and 3 tablespoons of the juice from the tomatoes in a small saucepan and saute until vegetables soften. Add the tomatoes. Simmer for 30 to 40 minutes until thickened. (This recipe makes 3 cups, with 33 calories per ½ cup.)

Gazpacho

Makes 6 servings (64 calories each)

1½ cups peeled chopped tomatoes
  1 cup chopped red or green
    sweet peppers
  2 cups peeled, seeded and
    chopped cucumbers
  1 cup chopped Spanish onion
  1 clove garlic, minced
  1 tablespoon chopped fresh
    parsley
  1 tablespoon chopped fresh
    basil or 1½ teaspoons
    dried basil
  1 tablespoon chopped fresh
    chervil (optional)
  pinch of cayenne pepper
  1 tablespoon tamari or soy
    sauce
  ½ teaspoon black pepper
  3 cups tomato juice or water
    lemon slices (garnish)
    parsley sprigs (garnish)

In a small bowl, reserve ½ cup tomatoes, ⅓ cup peppers, ⅔ cup cucumbers and ⅓ cup onions.

Place the remaining tomatoes, peppers, cucumbers and onions, the garlic, parsley, basil, chervil (if used), tamari or soy sauce, pepper and tomato juice or water in food processor or blender and puree until very smooth. Pour puree into a large ceramic or glass bowl and stir in reserved ingredients. Cover bowl and chill until ready to serve.

Garnish with thin slices of lemon and/or sprigs of parsley.

Red Snapper with Salsa

Makes 4 servings (207 calories each)

1½ pounds red snapper
  ½ cup lime juice
  1 small red onion, coarsely
    chopped
  1 clove garlic, minced
  1 can (4 ounces) chopped green
    chili peppers
  1 can (16 ounces) tomatoes,
    drained and coarsely
    chopped, or 3 small
    fresh tomatoes, peeled,
    seeded and coarsely
    chopped
  ½ cup finely chopped fresh
    coriander leaves

Place fish in a glass or ceramic container, pour lime juice over it and cover. Marinate in the refrigerator for at least 2 hours.

To make the salsa, combine the remaining ingredients and mix well.

Drain fish and reserve the marinade. Arrange the fish in a baking dish large enough to hold it all in one layer. Mix half the marinade with the salsa and spread over top of the fish. Cover the baking dish with foil and bake in a preheated 350°F oven for 20 minutes, or until done (the baking time will vary, depending on the thickness of the fish fillets). Serve immediately.

Tostadas

Makes 6 tostadas (173 calories each)

  6 corn tortillas
  3 cups low-fat cottage cheese
  1 green chili pepper, minced
  2 tablespoons chopped pimiento
  1 shallot, minced
  ½ teaspoon chili powder
  ½ teaspoon tamari or soy sauce
  6 lettuce leaves
  1 tomato, chopped (garnish)
  ½ cup chopped green bell pepper
    (garnish)

Brush both sides of tortillas lightly with oil. Place on baking sheet and bake in a preheated 425°F oven for about 5 minutes, or until crisp and lightly browned.

In a medium bowl, combine the cottage cheese, chili peppers, pimiento, shallots, chili powder and tamari or soy sauce. Mix well and refrigerate for 1 hour to blend flavors.

To assemble, place a lettuce leaf on each tortilla and fill each with ½ cup of the cheese mixture. Garnish with tomatoes and peppers.

Gazpacho, Red Snapper
with Salsa and Tostadas

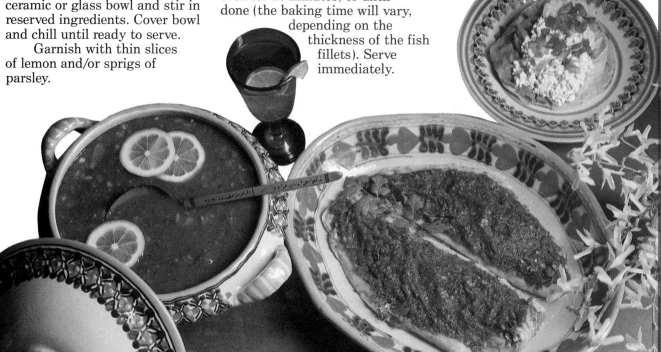

China

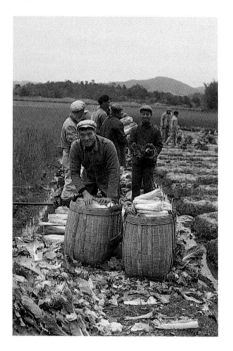

"The Chinese truly enjoy eating," says Sue Pai Yang, a registered dietitian from Livingston, New Jersey. "Eating is very important socially. That goes for Chinese-Americans, too. A gathering always means having a meal together—we don't invite people to come over just for cocktails. And Chinese cooking, of course, is regarded as a high form of art."

Nonetheless, "obesity is not a problem in China," Mrs. Yang states flatly. Her research in Beijing hospitals shows that the average Chinese eats between 2,000 and 3,000 calories a day—"90 percent of which is grains and vegetables."

On the other hand, Chinese-Americans are becoming more overweight than their relatives in China, she says. "As Chinese-Americans adopt American ways of eating, they eat more fat and meat and start having dessert after meals." And, she points out, "Chinese-Americans add more fat in cooking than do native Chinese."

Traditional steamed bread, for example, is very low in fat; it's just water, flour and yeast. (A typical American biscuit mix, on the other hand, calls for ½ cup of shortening.) Also, salad foods like cucumbers and sprouts are often marinated in a sauce of vinegar, soy sauce and perhaps a drop of sesame oil—it has practically no calories to speak of. Vegetables aren't draped in cream sauces, but are steamed or lightly sauteed to retain nutrients and make the most of fresh, natural flavors and textures.

All of which is a good argument for eating the way the Chinese *in China* do. To help you get acquainted with the Chinese way of eating, we offer you these traditional dishes, all low in fat and calories.

Hot-and-Sour Soup

Makes 6 servings (112 calories each)

4 dried black mushrooms
2 cups warm water
5 cups chicken stock
¼ pound boned skinned chicken breast (about ½ breast), slivered
¼ cup slivered bamboo shoots
¼ pound firm tofu, cut into ⅛-inch cubes
3 tablespoons rice vinegar
1 tablespoon tamari or soy sauce
hot pepper sauce, to taste
¼ teaspoon freshly ground black pepper
2 tablespoons cornstarch
¼ cup water

1 egg, beaten
2 teaspoons sesame oil
1 scallion, thinly sliced and separated into rings (garnish)

In a medium bowl, soak the dried mushrooms in the warm water for 30 minutes. Drain and reserve 1 cup soaking liquid. Sliver the mushrooms.

In a large saucepan, combine the stock and mushroom soaking liquid and bring to a boil over medium-high heat. Add the chicken, bamboo shoots and mushrooms. Bring to a boil, then reduce heat and simmer, covered, for 10 minutes. Add tofu and simmer, covered, for 3 minutes longer. Stir in the vinegar, tamari or soy sauce, hot pepper sauce and pepper.

In a small bowl, stir the cornstarch and water together to form a paste. Stir into hot soup and cook to thicken, 1 or 2 minutes.

Gently stir in the egg and oil. Remove from heat. Sprinkle with scallions.

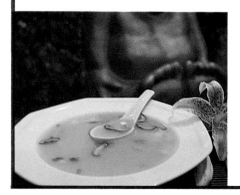

Ginger-Mushroom Fish Fillets

Makes 6 servings (149 calories each)

⅓ cup chopped scallions
1¼ cup thinly sliced mushrooms
1 tablespoon tamari or soy sauce
½ to ¾ teaspoon grated peeled ginger root
1 teaspoon lemon juice
¼ cup chicken stock or fish stock
1½ pounds fish fillets, such as sole or flounder

In a medium bowl, mix the scallions, mushrooms, tamari or soy sauce, ginger and lemon juice.

Heat the stock in a large skillet. The liquid should barely cover the bottom of the pan. Place the fish in the pan, being careful not to overlap the pieces. Spread the mushroom mixture over the fish immediately. Cover and simmer 5 to 7 minutes.

Be very careful that the fish does not overcook; as soon as it flakes, it is done. Remove from heat and serve immediately, accompanied by brown rice, if desired.

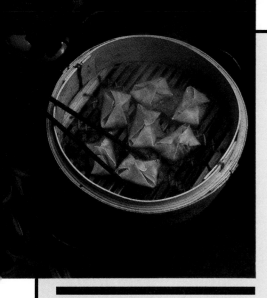

Steamed Dumplings with Dipping Sauce

Makes 24 dumplings (43 calories each)

In Chinese cuisine, dumplings are often fried. The steaming method used here cuts calories without cutting the flavor.

⅔ cup (about ¼ pound) minced cooked chicken
¼ cup chopped cooked spinach
¼ cup mashed tofu
1 tablespoon chopped scallions
4 tablespoons plus 1 teaspoon tamari or soy sauce
1 teaspoon rice vinegar
2 teaspoons apple juice
1 to 2 teaspoons minced peeled ginger root
24 wonton wrappers
1 tablespoon sesame oil
Dipping Sauce

In a medium bowl, combine the chicken, spinach, tofu, scallions, 1 tablespoon plus 1 teaspoon tamari or soy sauce, vinegar, apple juice and ginger. Drop by teaspoons onto wonton wrappers and fold.

In a 1-quart ovenproof casserole, stir together 1 tablespoon tamari or soy sauce and 1 teaspoon oil. Place 8 dumplings in the dish and place on a steaming rack. Cover and place over boiling water. Cook until dumplings steam, about 10 to 15 minutes.

Remove, wrap in foil and place in a warm oven. Repeat steaming process until all dumplings are cooked.

Prepare sauce as dumplings steam.

DIPPING SAUCE

1 tablespoon cornstarch
2 tablespoons tamari or soy sauce
1 cup water
dash of Tabasco sauce
2 teaspoons apricot jelly
½ teaspoon honey
2 cloves garlic, minced

In a small saucepan, combine the cornstarch and tamari or soy sauce to form a liquid paste. Slowly whisk in the water, then place over medium-high heat. Whisking constantly, add the Tabasco, jelly, honey and garlic. Cook until syrupy.

Pour into small bowls and serve with dumplings. (This recipe makes about ¼ cup, with 9 calories per teaspoon.)

Oven-Crisped Egg Rolls

Makes 8 egg rolls (148 calories each)

Unnecessary calories can be eliminated by baking instead of deep frying these Oriental favorites.

¼ pound boned skinned chicken breast (about ½ breast), slivered
1 tablespoon plus 1 teaspoon tamari or soy sauce
5 to 6 tablespoons chicken stock
2 scallions, minced
1 cup shredded Chinese cabbage
1 cup finely chopped broccoli florets
1 cup mung bean sprouts
½ cup slivered bamboo shoots
¼ cup slivered water chestnuts
8 egg roll wrappers
1 egg, beaten
1 tablespoon vegetable oil

In a small bowl, toss together the chicken and 1 teaspoon tamari or soy sauce. Let stand for 10 minutes.

Place 3 tablespoons of stock in a large skillet and bring to a boil over medium-high heat. Add the chicken and cook, stirring constantly, until chicken is no longer pink, about 2 minutes. Remove chicken from pan and set aside.

Add 2 tablespoons stock to the pan and heat it. Add the scallions, cabbage and broccoli and cook, stirring constantly, for about 2 minutes. If necessary, add remaining tablespoon of stock to pan to prevent sticking. Add the bean sprouts, bamboo shoots and water chestnuts and cook, stirring constantly, for 1 minute. Add remaining tamari or soy sauce and the chicken and blend. Remove from heat.

Drain filling in a colander if necessary and allow to cool. Make sure the filling is dry.

Place ⅓ cup filling on each egg roll wrapper and fold. Brush the edges of each egg roll with beaten egg to help seal it, then brush each with a small amount of the oil.

Spray a baking sheet with nonstick spray, then place the egg rolls on the baking sheet and bake in a preheated 450°F oven for 6 minutes, then turn and bake another 6 minutes, until lightly browned.

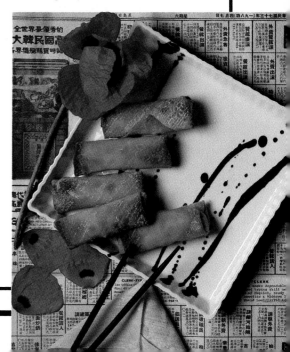

Japan

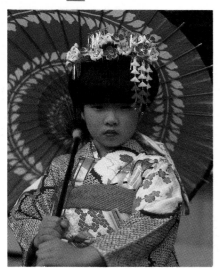

In the subways of Tokyo at rush hour, you can't count the multitude of people, but you *can* count the number of chubby Japanese—on one hand. How do they stay so slim? Various factors count. First of all, they eat a low-fat diet—14 to 23 percent of their daily intake comes from fats, most of them polyunsaturated. They eat a lot of rice and soy products: Carbohydrates comprise 58 to 65 percent of the diet. They eat far more fish and shellfish than meat.

On top of that, when Mama-san serves a meal "family style," that means she's divvied up vegetables and fish among family members and placed them artistically in small, attractive dishes. Rice is eaten between mouthfuls of other food, not all at once, and is treated almost reverently: Children are taught early to always receive the rice bowl with both hands, and not to leave a grain behind unless they want seconds. A mouthful left at the bottom of the bowl subtly says, "More rice, please."

Also, deep down, the Japanese believe it's virtuous to leave the table a little bit hungry. And they are aghast at the idea of eating while standing or walking outside, except under very specific circumstances (such as the stand-up McDonald's food bar on the Ginza, where one eats "American-style").

Scientists agree that those eating habits have paid off health-wise, in a lowered incidence of obesity and obesity-related disorders such as heart disease. So, take a tip from the Japanese and indulge yourself in their delightful cuisine.

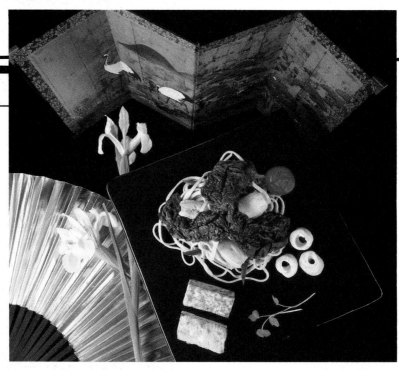

Chicken Sukiyaki

Makes 6 servings (469 calories each)

½ pound dried whole wheat udon noodles
12 pieces dried wheat gluten, 1 inch square
¼ cup tamari or soy sauce
1 cup chicken stock
3 tablespoons honey
1 pound tofu, cut into 2- by 1-inch rectangles
1 chicken (broiler-fryer, 3 pounds), skinned, boned and cut into 2- by 1-inch pieces
12 scallions, sliced diagonally into 2-inch pieces
4 ounces fresh spinach, stems removed

Cook noodles, drain, rinse in cold running water and set aside. Soak wheat gluten in tepid water until soft, about 15 minutes. Drain, squeeze out excess water and set aside.

Place tamari or soy sauce, ½ cup stock and honey in a medium saucepan. Bring to a boil over medium heat, stirring frequently. Remove from heat and set aside. Broil the tofu, turning to brown on all sides.

Lightly coat a large, heavy skillet with oil. In the skillet bring the remaining ½ cup stock to a boil and add the chicken and tofu. Cook over high heat for 2 minutes, stirring frequently. Remove from heat.

Using a slotted spoon, transfer the chicken and tofu from the skillet and add to the soy sauce mixture. Allow to soak for 5 minutes. Return the chicken and tofu to the skillet and stir-fry over high heat. Add, in this order, the soy sauce mixture, scallions, noodles and wheat gluten. Stir-fry until liquid evaporates. Add the spinach and stir-fry until it is wilted.

NOTE: Thick, eggless whole wheat udon noodles are available in Oriental food stores.

Chicken with Noodles in Broth

Makes 4 servings (180 calories each)

 5 cups light chicken stock
 1 pound boned skinned chicken breast (about 2 breasts)
¼ cup chopped scallions
 1 tablespoon tamari or soy sauce
 3 teaspoons chopped peeled ginger root
 6 Sichuan peppercorns
 1 cup (about 2½ ounces) whole wheat pasta or buckwheat pasta
 1 tablespoon sesame oil
¼ teaspoon Tabasco sauce
 2 tablespoons chopped scallions (garnish)

Bring the stock to a boil in a 3- to 4-quart pot. Add the chicken, scallions, tamari or soy sauce, ginger and peppercorns. Reduce heat to medium-low and poach chicken in barely simmering stock until tender, 10 to 15 minutes. Remove chicken from stock and shred. Strain stock and return to pot.

Cook the pasta in boiling water according to package directions. Drain. Add pasta, shredded chicken, oil and Tabasco to warm stock and stir to heat through. Ladle into four warmed serving bowls. Sprinkle with scallions and serve.

Buckwheat Noodles with Vegetables in Spicy Sauce

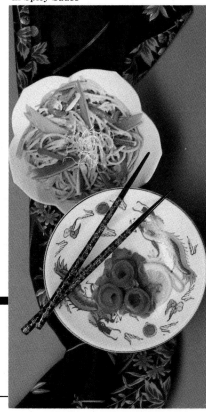

Buckwheat Noodles and Vegetables in Spicy Sauce

Makes 4 servings (348 calories each)

¼ pound snow peas
 1 small green or red pepper, cut into ⅛-inch strips
 1 small zucchini, cut into ⅛-inch julienne strips
¼ cup peanut butter or sesame butter
½ cup strong chicken stock or vegetable stock
½ teaspoon Tabasco sauce
 1 tablespoon tamari or soy sauce
 1 tablespoon rice vinegar
 8 ounces buckwheat noodles or thin whole wheat noodles
 2 tablespoons chopped scallions
½ cup alfalfa sprouts (garnish)

Remove the strings from the snow peas, then mix with the peppers and zucchini in a large bowl.

To prepare the sauce, place the peanut or sesame butter, stock, Tabasco, tamari or soy sauce, vinegar and scallions in a food processor or blender and process until smooth.

Cook the noodles in boiling water according to package directions. Drain. While still hot, toss with vegetables and sauce.

Marinate in the refrigerator overnight to allow flavors to blend. To serve, divide into four portions and top with sprouts.

Miso Soup

Makes 4 servings (70 calories each)

 4 shiitake mushrooms
 4 cups water
 2 scallions
½ cup snow peas
 1 4-inch section kombu (optional)
 1 carrot, thinly sliced
¼ pound tofu, cubed
 2 tablespoons miso, any red or brown type

Soak mushrooms in 1 cup water until softened, about 20 minutes. Reserve the soaking liquid. Remove stems from mushrooms and cut the caps into bite-size pieces.

Thinly slice the scallions, keeping the white and green parts separate. Remove the strings from the snow peas. Place the remaining 3 cups water, the kombu (if used) and carrots in a large saucepan and bring to a boil. Remove and discard kombu as soon as it softens. When carrots are almost tender, reduce heat and add the snow peas, tofu, mushrooms and white parts of the scallions. Simmer 3 minutes.

Meanwhile, in a medium bowl, stir the mushroom soaking liquid into the miso to make a smooth, shiny paste. Add most of the miso to the soup and taste. Add more if desired. Keep soup just below a simmer for 4 minutes. (Do not allow soup to boil after miso is added.)

Serve hot, garnished with the scallion greens.

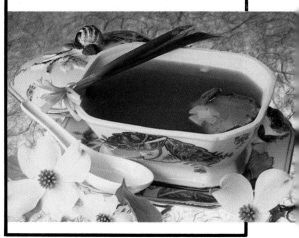

The Middle East

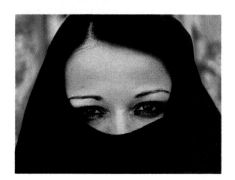

Hummus and *baba ghannouj* are but two Middle Eastern foods "making it" on the American food scene today. *Shish kabab*—skewered pieces of marinated meat (usually lamb) and vegetables—have long been on the menu at backyard barbecues. *Pita* bread has become so popular—even appearing at fast food restaurants—that people have begun to forget its Arabic origins.

If you patronize natural foods restaurants, chances are you'll run into pita "pockets," or pita-bread sandwiches filled with raw vegetables and cheese, tuna salad or *falafel*, an aromatic mashed-chick-pea patty.

Middle Eastern foods such as *tahini* and olive oil, *bulgur*, rice, dried apricots, yogurt and pine nuts are common items in many health food stores. It's no accident, either. The dishes native to Lebanon, Syria, Iran and Turkey tend to be naturally low in saturated fats, high in nutrients and fiber and generally good for your body and your palate.

Meat, mostly lamb, is used sparingly. *Kibbeh* is a classic meat dish of pounded lamb mixed with bulgur, pine nuts and allspice. In some traditions, olive oil practically drenches the food. By preparing Middle Eastern foods at home, you can drastically cut back on excess oil. The essential flavor won't be affected at all.

Shish Taouk

Makes 4 servings (203 calories each)

The marinade for this dish is made with yogurt rather than oil.

3 tablespoons fresh lemon juice
1 cup low-fat yogurt
4 cloves garlic, crushed
½ teaspoon paprika
1 teaspoon minced fresh mint or
    ½ teaspoon crushed dried
    mint
1 pound boned skinned chicken
    breast (about 2 breasts),
    cut into 2-inch cubes
8 large mushrooms
2 green peppers, cut into 1-inch
    pieces

In a medium bowl, whisk together the lemon juice, yogurt, garlic, paprika and mint. Add chicken and mushrooms and toss gently, coating well. Marinate in refrigerator 8 hours or overnight.

Place chicken, mushrooms and peppers on four 12-inch skewers. Broil until golden brown, about 10 minutes on each side.

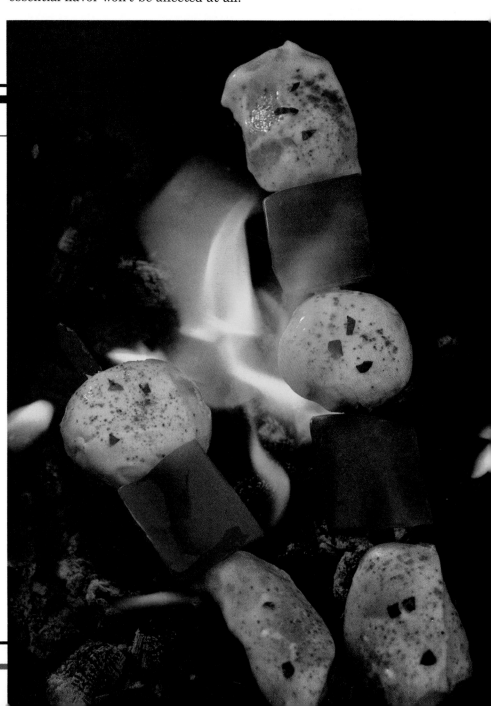

Falafel

Makes 20 patties (75 calories each)

Fried to a crisp coat, this regional version absorbs little oil.

½ pound dried white fava
    beans, soaked 24 hours
2 tablespoons sesame tahini
2½ to 3 teaspoons ground cumin
½ teaspoon ground turmeric
2 to 3 cloves garlic, minced
1 teaspoon ground coriander
2 tablespoons chopped fresh
    parsley
1 egg, slightly beaten
1½ scallions, chopped
2 tablespoons whole wheat
    bread crumbs
dash of cayenne pepper
2 to 3 tablespoons olive oil

Remove skins from beans, then place beans in a food processor and puree to a smooth paste, or mash by hand.

In a medium bowl, combine the bean paste, tahini, herbs and spices, egg, scallions, bread crumbs and cayenne. Cover and refrigerate 1 hour. Shape into patties 2 inches in diameter. Let rest 15 minutes.

In a large skillet, heat 1 tablespoon oil until hot. Fry 10 patties until brown, about 2 minutes on each side. Remove. Add 1 tablespoon oil to skillet and repeat with remaining patties. Serve with pita bread.

Imam Bayildi

Makes 4 servings (199 calories each)

To cut calories, the eggplant is baked in water instead of simmered in oil.

2 medium eggplants
  juice of 3 lemons
2 tablespoons olive oil
1 medium onion, thinly sliced
¼ cup sliced mushrooms
¼ cup chopped parsley
4 cups peeled chopped tomatoes
  freshly grated nutmeg, to taste
½ cup water

Cut the eggplants in half lengthwise. Scoop out flesh, dice it and place in a small bowl.

Pour lemon juice over eggplant shells and flesh. Let stand 30 minutes, then drain.

Heat 1 tablespoon oil in a medium skillet. Add diced eggplant, onions and mushrooms. Saute until tender, 5 to 7 minutes.

In a medium bowl, combine the vegetables, parsley, tomatoes and nutmeg. Place this mixture in the eggplant shells. Place filled shells in a 9 × 11-inch baking pan. Brush top of filling with remaining oil. Pour water into bottom of pan. Cover and bake in a preheated 350°F oven until tender, 25 to 30 minutes.

Remove from oven and chill. Serve cold.

Pita Sandwich

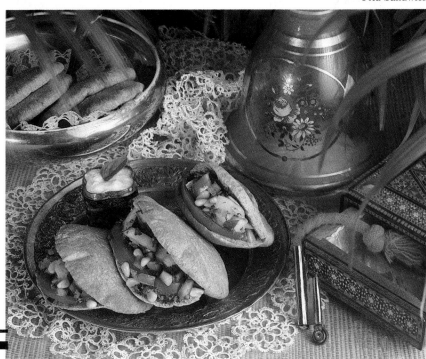

Pita Sandwich

Makes 4 servings (299 calories each)

1⅓ cup diced cucumber
2 medium tomatoes, sliced
1 large Italian frying pepper,
    seeded and diced
2 tablespoons chopped fresh
    parsley

1 tablespoon pine nuts or
    chopped walnuts
¼ cup sesame tahini
½ cup low-fat yogurt
½ cup fresh lemon juice
2 cloves garlic, minced
½ teaspoon minced fresh mint
    or ¼ teaspoon crushed
    dried mint
4 pita pockets

In a medium bowl, gently toss together the cucumbers, tomatoes, peppers, parsley and nuts. In a small bowl, whisk together the tahini, yogurt, lemon juice, garlic and mint. Pour over vegetables and toss gently until well coated. Chill 1 hour. Spoon into pita bread and serve.

Greece

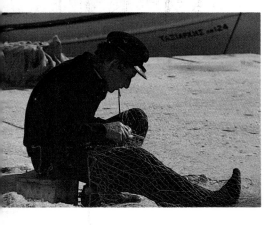

The Greeks make full use of their Mediterranean gifts: olives and lemons from groves on the hillsides; tomatoes and cucumbers, eggplant and okra that flourish in the sunny clime; squid and fish from the azure sea. The goats that climb the rocky slopes provide milk, cheese and yogurt. Sheep grazing in open fields give a delicious creamy yogurt. Lamb is the Greeks' favorite meat. Onion and garlic flavor many dishes, and a touch of cinnamon adds a Greek piquancy to any tomato sauce.

Greek cooking can't be called haute cuisine, but the Greeks have a knack for making the most out of simple foodstuffs. Greece "was never a rich source of food," writes James Trager in *The Foodbook*. "Less than a quarter of its land can be tilled." Perhaps that's why the Greeks don't seem to give a second thought to calories—an overabundance of food was never their "problem." But we have given thought to the calories and offer you some lighter versions of traditional Greek dishes and some that are naturally low in calories.

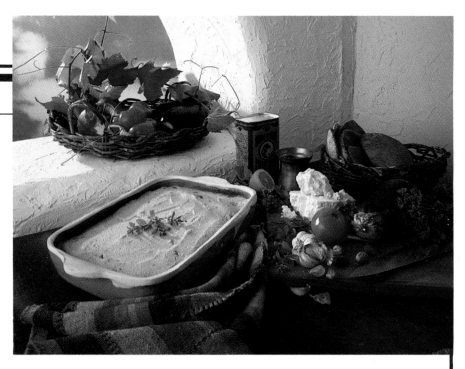

Moussaka

Makes 6 servings (234 calories each)

Less meat and oil are used in this dish to cut calories and fat.

1 medium eggplant
  juice of 1 lemon
1 teaspoon olive oil
1 medium onion, chopped
2 cloves garlic, minced
½ cup sliced mushrooms
¼ pound lean ground beef
¾ cup mashed tofu
¾ cup tomato sauce
¼ cup water
1 tablespoon white wine
  vinegar
3 tablespoons apple juice
2 tablespoons chopped fresh
  parsley
2 tablespoons crumbled feta
  cheese
1 teaspoon minced fresh
  oregano or ½ teaspoon
  crushed dried oregano
  freshly ground black pepper
1 egg, separated
2 tablespoons dry whole wheat
  bread crumbs
1⅓ cups milk
⅓ cup cornmeal
2 tablespoons butter
1 teaspoon grated nutmeg
2 teaspoons Parmesan cheese

Cut the eggplant lengthwise into ½-inch slices. Squeeze lemon juice over the slices and soak 30 minutes, then drain. Broil the slices until lightly browned, 2 or 3 minutes on each side. Set aside.

Heat the oil in a large skillet. Add the onions, garlic and mushrooms. Saute until tender, about 5 minutes. Add the meat and cook until browned, about 10 minutes. Stir in the tofu, tomato sauce, water, vinegar and apple juice. Simmer 5 minutes.

In a medium bowl, combine the sauteed mixture with the parsley, feta, oregano, pepper and egg white.

Lightly grease an 8 × 8 × 2-inch pan. Sprinkle bread crumbs on the bottom and sides of pan. Spread half the eggplant on the bottom of the pan, then spread half the meat mixture over the eggplant. Repeat with remaining eggplant and meat.

In a small saucepan, whisk together the milk and cornmeal. Add the butter and whisk over medium heat until hot. Lightly beat the egg yolk in a small bowl. Whisk in ¼ cup milk mixture, then quickly whisk this mixture back into remaining milk. Whisking constantly, cook until thickened, 3 to 5 minutes. Stir in nutmeg and Parmesan cheese.

Pour the milk mixture into the pan. Bake in a preheated 375°F oven until golden, about 25 minutes.

Spanakopita (Greek Spinach Pie)

Makes 4 servings (323 calories each)

Calories are saved in this dish by replacing some feta cheese with cottage cheese and tofu.

3 tablespoons butter
¼ cup chopped onion
2 cloves garlic, minced
2 cups chopped cooked spinach
2 cups low-fat cottage cheese
1 egg
½ cup mashed tofu
2 tablespoons crumbled feta cheese
½ teaspoon ground nutmeg
3 tablespoons bread crumbs
6 sheets phyllo pastry

Melt 1 tablespoon butter in a medium skillet. Add the onions and garlic and saute until tender, about 3 minutes.

In a large bowl, combine the onions, garlic, spinach, cottage cheese, egg, tofu, feta and nutmeg.

Melt the remaining butter in a small saucepan. Lightly brush the bottom and sides of an 8 × 8 × 2-inch baking pan with the butter. Sprinkle the bottom with 1 tablespoon bread crumbs.

Cut the phyllo in half widthwise. Place 1 cut piece in the pan and sprinkle with 1 teaspoon bread crumbs. Place another piece on top of the first and brush with 1 teaspoon butter. Repeat the sequence with two more pieces of phyllo. Spread the spinach mixture evenly on the phyllo. Cover with 1 piece of phyllo and sprinkle with 1 teaspoon bread crumbs. Place another piece on top and brush with 1 teaspoon butter. Repeat sequence with the remaining two pieces of phyllo.

Cut the spanakopita diago-

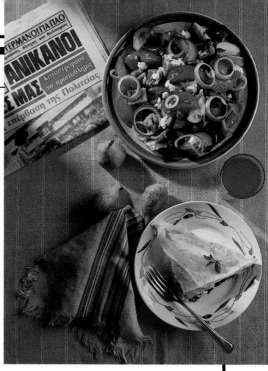

Greek Salata and Spanakopita

nally to form four triangles. Bake in a preheated 350°F oven until golden, about 20 minutes. Allow to cool 10 to 15 minutes before removing from pan.

Avgolemono Soup (Greek Chicken–Lemon Soup)

Makes 4 servings (106 calories each)

Calorie-conscious Greek women eat this for lunch.

4 cups chicken stock
1 tablespoon fresh lemon juice
¼ teaspoon grated lemon rind
½ cup cooked brown rice
4 egg yolks, slightly beaten
  freshly ground black pepper
  freshly ground nutmeg

Heat stock in a 2-quart saucepan until steaming. Stir in lemon juice and rind. Add rice and heat.

Whisk ¼ cup of stock into egg yolks, then quickly whisk mixture back into stock. Heat gently, stirring occasionally, until steaming, 2 to 3 minutes.

Pour into serving bowls and sprinkle with pepper and nutmeg.

Zadziki (Cucumber – Yogurt Salad)

Makes 4 servings (111 calories each)

2 cups low-fat yogurt
2 to 3 cloves garlic, crushed
1 tablespoon white wine vinegar or lemon juice
1 tablespoon olive oil
2 cups chopped cucumbers

In a medium bowl, whisk together the yogurt, garlic, vinegar or lemon juice and oil. Stir in the cucumbers. Chill at least 1 hour or overnight. Serve over a bed of romaine lettuce with pita bread.

Zadziki

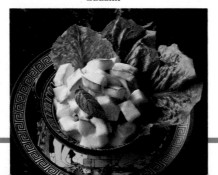

Greek Salata

Makes 4 servings (192 calories each)

2 tomatoes, quartered
1 large cucumber, halved and cut into ¼-inch slices
2 green peppers or Italian frying peppers, seeded and diced
¼ cup broken walnuts
⅓ cup crumbled feta cheese
1 small sweet onion, sliced and separated into rings
2 tablespoons olive oil
⅓ cup fresh lemon juice
2 teaspoons minced fresh oregano or 1 teaspoon crushed dried oregano
1 clove garlic, crushed

In a medium bowl, gently toss the tomatoes, cucumbers, peppers, walnuts, feta and onions. In a separate bowl, whisk together the oil, lemon juice, oregano and garlic. Pour dressing over vegetables and toss gently. Refrigerate 1 hour before serving.

Eastern Europe

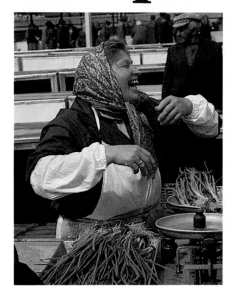

Beneath the wide umbrella of Eastern European cookery are the cuisines of Poland, the USSR, East Germany, Czechoslovakia, Hungary, Romania, Bulgaria, Yugoslavia and Albania. While each cuisine has its distinctive taste, all base their dishes on many of the same ingredients: noodles and dumplings, sour cream and cottage-type cheeses, sausages, cabbage rolls stuffed with meat and rice, meat stews *(goulashes)*, buckwheat groats *(kasha)* and *pilaf* and butter-rich pastries and tortes.

Borscht (a soup most often found in Jewish delicatessens in the U.S.) is a good example of a food that crosses boundaries. In *The Best of Ethnic Home Cooking,* Mary Poulos Wilde writes, "Eastern European in origin, borscht simply is a healthful, deep claret-colored soup based on fresh beets which is served hot or cold. The similarities end here. Certain kinds of borscht are creamy with the addition of a frothy egg whisked into the bubbling broth. Other versions feature a steaming hot boiled potato without the jacket drenched with ice cold beet broth and mounded with thick sour cream. What's more, this fragrant soup changes with the addition of chopped egg, chopped and seeded cucumber, chives, lemon rind, and even tiny shrimp."

Humble in origin, this cuisine is so flexible it offers a whole range of taste pleasures for those seeking lighter fare. You'll find through our recipes that it's easy to use low-calorie substitutes for high-calorie ingredients in many dishes.

Chicken Paprikash

Makes 6 servings (284 calories each)

Yogurt replaces high-calorie sour cream in this Hungarian favorite.

2 pounds boned skinned chicken breast (about 4 breasts)
2 onions, thinly sliced
5 teaspoons Hungarian paprika
1 cup water
2 teaspoons tamari or soy sauce
¼ to ½ teaspoon black pepper

1 tablespoon whole wheat pastry flour
½ cup low-fat yogurt

Place the chicken breasts in a large, heavy saucepan. In a medium bowl, combine the onions, paprika, water, tamari or soy sauce and black pepper and pour over chicken. Cover and cook over medium heat for 30 to 40 minutes, or until chicken is tender. Remove chicken, place on a serving platter, cover and keep warm.

In a small bowl, whisk the flour into the yogurt. Add yogurt mixture to the juices in the pan and gradually bring to a boil, stirring constantly. The liquid will be thin and yogurt may appear curdled at first. Continue to boil and stir until sauce has thickened and yogurt is smooth. Remove from heat and pour over chicken.

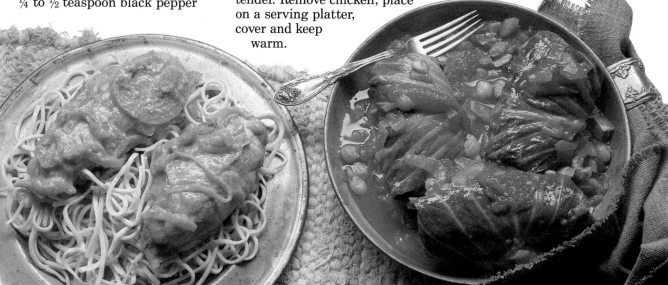

Chicken Paprikash and Stuffed Cabbage

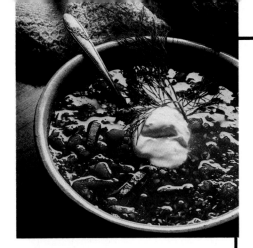

Stuffed Cabbage

Makes 14 cabbage rolls (101 calories each)

Tofu replaces part of the ground beef to lessen the saturated fat in this dish.

1 large head cabbage
2 medium onions, finely chopped
3 cups tomatoes, peeled and crushed
½ cup tomato puree
1 to 2 teaspoons tamari or soy sauce
¼ to ½ teaspoon black pepper
½ cup chopped golden raisins
½ pound lean ground beef
½ pound tofu, crumbled
1 egg
¼ cup cooked brown rice
1 clove garlic, minced

Place the cabbage in a large, deep, heat-resistant container. Add enough boiling water to cover. Soak for 15 minutes, drain and repeat as often as necessary to soften leaves.

Place the onions, tomatoes, tomato puree, tamari or soy sauce, pepper and raisins in a large, deep saucepan. Cover and simmer for 30 minutes.

In a medium bowl, mix together the beef, tofu, egg, rice and garlic. Gently remove a leaf from the cabbage. Place about 2 tablespoons of the beef mixture onto it and roll, folding the sides in. Secure with a toothpick, if necessary. Continue until all stuffing is used.

Gently place rolls into tomato sauce. Baste with sauce, cover and simmer, basting occasionally, for 2 hours, or until tender.

Borscht

Makes 10 servings (81 calories each)

Traditional borscht is generally not pureed. However, this thicker, rich-tasting version, although still low in calories, may be more satisfying to a weight watcher as a one-dish meal.

1 cup chopped onions
½ cup chopped carrots
2½ cups chopped potatoes
1 teaspoon caraway seeds
1 teaspoon dillweed
4 cups vegetable stock or water
4 cups finely shredded cabbage
1 can (16 ounces) julienned salt-free beets, with juice

Place the onions, carrots, potatoes, caraway seeds, dill and 2 cups of stock or water in a kettle or stockpot. Simmer for 7 to 10 minutes, until the vegetables are barely tender. Add the cabbage and the remaining 2 cups of stock or water. Cook over medium-low heat for approximately 10 minutes, until cabbage is cooked.

With a slotted spoon, put about half of the cooked vegetables in a blender with enough vegetable water to puree them easily. Return pureed vegetables to pot with any remaining stock. Stir in beets and beet juice. Simmer just long enough to heat all ingredients. Serve hot or cold with a dollop of yogurt.

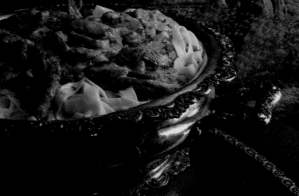

Beef and Mushroom Stroganoff

Makes 4 servings (488 calories each)

Yogurt replaces the sour cream in this Russian national dish.

1 pound beef sirloin, cut into ¼-inch strips
3 tablespoons whole wheat flour
1 tablespoon vegetable oil
1 pound mushrooms, sliced
½ cup finely chopped onion
1 clove garlic, minced
1 teaspoon dried tarragon
1 teaspoon tamari or soy sauce
1¼ cups beef stock
1 cup yogurt

Coat meat with 1 tablespoon of the flour. Heat the oil in a skillet, then add the meat and brown quickly on both sides. Add the mushrooms, onions, garlic and tarragon and cook over medium heat for 3 to 5 minutes. Using a slotted spoon, remove meat and mushrooms from pan. Set aside.

Brown remaining flour in pan drippings. Add tamari or soy sauce and stock. Stir over medium heat until thick and bubbly. Spoon some hot sauce into yogurt and blend well, then add yogurt to pan and stir well. Return meat and mushrooms to pan and cook over low heat 2 to 3 minutes, until heated through; do not boil. Serve over hot noodles or rice, if desired.

4

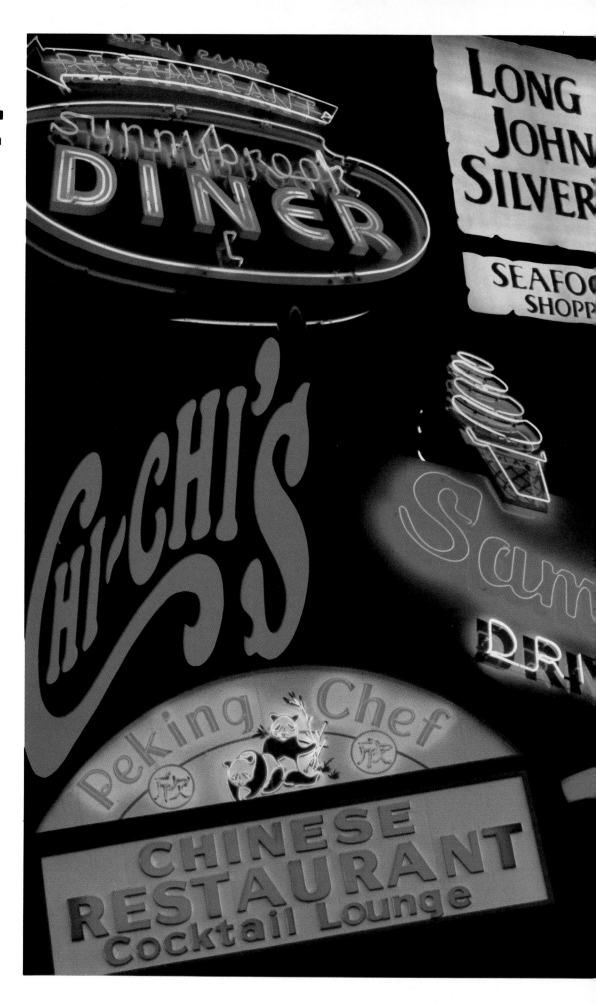

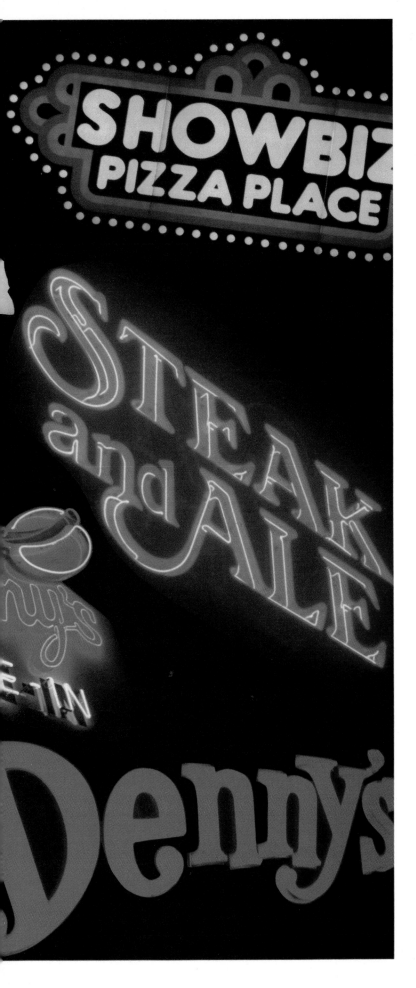

The Fine Art of Dining Out

Eating in a restaurant needn't be a liability in your efforts to control your weight.

Gordon took good restaurant reviews as literally as some folks take the Bible, and he often quoted them line by line the way a preacher might the Holy Book. But his fervor got Gordon into trouble. The 45-year-old Southerner, a traveling salesman, clipped dozens of reviews from out-of-town newspapers, saved them in his wallet and, when he passed through an unfamiliar city, made it a point to try an establishment featured in one of his clippings. Unfortunately, he often felt compelled to try almost all of the foods listed in the reviews. If one touted the "crusty garlic bread, dripping with butter and oozing with Parmesan cheese," Gordon ate several pieces of it. And, oh, the desserts! When a reviewer bragged of trying a piece of "heavenly, melt-in-your-mouth chocolate-almond torte" or "sponge cake, swimming in Grand Marnier sauce and topped with whipped cream and flecks of coconut," Gordon tried both.

Thus, Gordon's love affair with great restaurants added up, much the way the reviews piled up—he became 100 pounds overweight. When he finally checked in to a weight-control clinic, one of the first things his doctor did was put Gordon's reviews in a pile and set it on fire.

Of course, not everyone has to take such drastic actions to lose weight. But Gordon's dilemma mirrors that of many in modern society who regard eating out as a sort of mini-vacation from the rules. For many people, "dine out" and "pig out" are interchangeable terms.

Gerard Musante, Ph.D., who operates Structure House, a weight-control center in Durham, North Carolina, where Gordon went for help, says that eating out can be a "serious problem" for many trying to control their weight because it is regarded as a situation in which "control just doesn't exist."

And the fact that eating out is a big part of the American way of life doesn't help the problem either. The average American household spends $28.21 eating 21 percent of its weekly meals away from home, with more than half of these meals eaten in full service or fast food restaurants. And the inducements can be seen everywhere.

EATING OUT— AN AMERICAN PASTIME

Newspapers and magazines in cities herald new restaurant openings by the score, featuring everything from Chinese and Middle Eastern to North African cuisines. There are few urban landscapes without a flickering neon "fast food row," beckoning diners to gorge on burgers, french fries, "thick" shakes and other body-bulging treats. And all this attention to food and dining out is given with little regard for the waistline.

One recent Gallup poll found that 6 out of every 10 American adults reported they have changed their eating habits at home for the better, either by eating more fruits, vegetables or whole grains, or by decreasing their consumption of refined sugar, animal fats or salt. However, when asked about their habits while eating out, many told an entirely different story. Only 4 out of 10 said they practiced the same good habits when dining out. And of those who had changed their habits, only 2 percent said they made an effort to cut calories while dining out.

Why? Because, as Dr. Musante explains, people regard eating out as an "escape from routine"—an occasion to suspend all rules.

DINING OUT ON A DIET CAN BE EASY

Does this mean that those who want to shed pounds or at least stay at the same level have to avoid restaurants the way a chronic gambler has to be sure not to set foot in a casino? Quite the contrary. It is very possible to lose weight *and* eat out, provided you arm yourself with a psychological game plan to deal with all the temptations. In fact, Dr. Musante has found that once people successfully learn some techniques, they discover that "restaurant meals are among the easiest to control."

Unfortunately, the obstacles for the uninitiated dining-out dieter are as varied as the menu itself. "If you tend to eat out a lot, it's very easy to gain weight because the dishes are often prepared with lots of butter, cream or cheese, or are swimming in calorie-filled sauces," says Andrea P. Boyar, Ph.D., a registered dietitian with the Mahoney Institute of the American Health Foundation, which has been encouraging restaurant chefs and owners to develop low-calorie gourmet food. In addition, restaurants are full of "food cues" that can derail even the most strong-willed weight watchers, says Dr. Musante. These include "the aromas from what other people are eating; the clinking of forks,

If you're an average American, your family eats 21 percent of its meals each week away from home. So says the most recent study conducted by National Family Opinion for *Restaurants & Institutions* magazine. As the chart shows, most of these away-from-home meals are lunch, followed by dinner, breakfast, snacks and brunch.

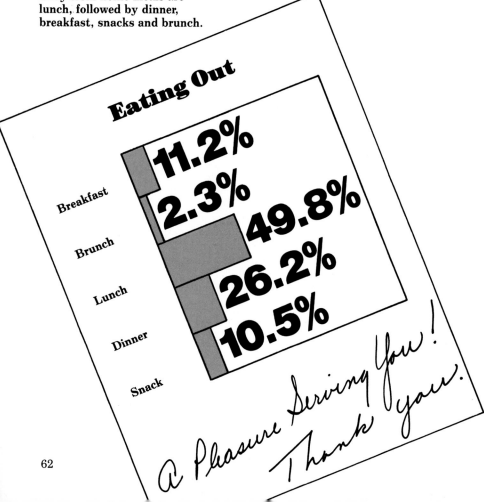

Eating Out

Breakfast **11.2%**

Brunch **2.3%**

Lunch **49.8%**

Dinner **26.2%**

Snack **10.5%**

A Pleasure Serving You! Thank you.

Watch This Fish Gain Weight

So you're going to play it safe and order fish at the restaurant tonight. If fish is on the menu, it can't be all that fattening, you reason to yourself. To find out how sound this reasoning is, we asked a seasoned chef to make a common restaurant specialty, stuffed flounder—a dish generally considered "safe" for the weight watcher. You may be surprised by what our camera and calculator came up with.

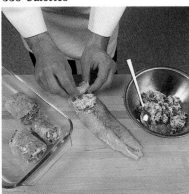

338 Calories

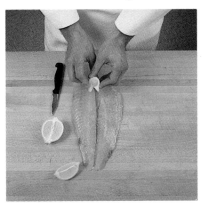

182 Calories

A half-pound of flounder at 179 calories and a bit of lemon wedge—not bad at all at 182 calories.

Now comes the stuffing—celery, scallions, parsley, red pepper and lemon juice, all at just over 4 calories; steamed crabmeat, at 15 calories; cracker crumbs (uh, oh) 38 calories; and a tablespoon of mayonnaise (oops!), 99 calories. But you're still okay at only 338 calories.

440 Calories

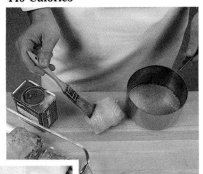

The fish is being broiled, not fried, so there's no need for butter or oil. Well, guess again. That generous brushing of butter and a dash of paprika just upped your calories by 102. You're now at 440 calories.

835 Calories

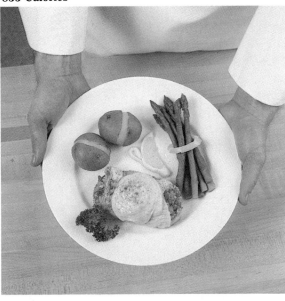

710 Calories

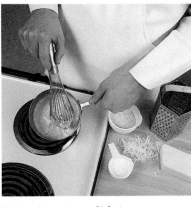

Hey, the menu didn't say anything about a sauce. Butter, flour, milk, cheese and heaven forbid, heavy cream—a total of 270 calories worth—and it's going to go all over your fish. You're now eating at the let-out-the-belt point—710 calories.

You can't expect to be served your fish on its own. A few boiled potatoes, stalks of asparagus and lemon wedges add another 125 calories to your meal. This "innocent" dining-out experience is costing you a total of 835 calories. The moral of this story? Don't be timid about asking your waiter or waitress lots of questions or even asking the chef to prepare it a special way—your way.

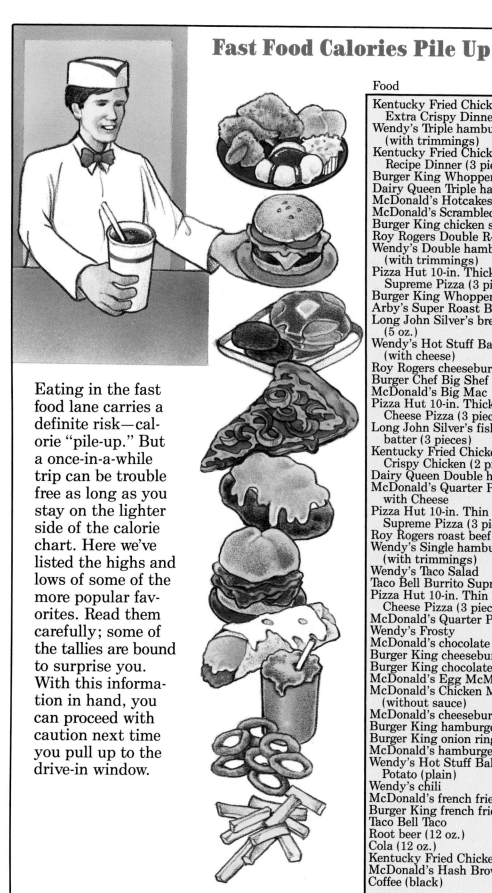

Fast Food Calories Pile Up

Eating in the fast food lane carries a definite risk—calorie "pile-up." But a once-in-a-while trip can be trouble free as long as you stay on the lighter side of the calorie chart. Here we've listed the highs and lows of some of the more popular favorites. Read them carefully; some of the tallies are bound to surprise you. With this information in hand, you can proceed with caution next time you pull up to the drive-in window.

Food	Calories
Kentucky Fried Chicken Extra Crispy Dinner (3 pieces)	950
Wendy's Triple hamburger (with trimmings)	850
Kentucky Fried Chicken Original Recipe Dinner (3 pieces)	830
Burger King Whopper with Cheese	740
Dairy Queen Triple hamburger	710
McDonald's Hotcakes and Sausage	706
McDonald's Scrambled Egg Breakfast	697
Burger King chicken sandwich	690
Roy Rogers Double R-Bar Burger	672
Wendy's Double hamburger (with trimmings)	670
Pizza Hut 10-in. Thick 'N Chewy Supreme Pizza (3 pieces)	640
Burger King Whopper	630
Arby's Super Roast Beef	620
Long John Silver's breaded clams (5 oz.)	617
Wendy's Hot Stuff Baked Potato (with cheese)	590
Roy Rogers cheeseburger	570
Burger Chef Big Shef	569
McDonald's Big Mac	563
Pizza Hut 10-in. Thick 'N Chewy Cheese Pizza (3 pieces)	560
Long John Silver's fish with batter (3 pieces)	549
Kentucky Fried Chicken Extra Crispy Chicken (2 pieces)	544
Dairy Queen Double hamburger	530
McDonald's Quarter Pounder with Cheese	524
Pizza Hut 10-in. Thin 'N Crispy Supreme Pizza (3 pieces)	510
Roy Rogers roast beef (large)	505
Wendy's Single hamburger (with trimmings)	470
Wendy's Taco Salad	460
Taco Bell Burrito Supreme	457
Pizza Hut 10-in. Thin 'N Crispy Cheese Pizza (3 pieces)	450
McDonald's Quarter Pounder	424
Wendy's Frosty	390
McDonald's chocolate shake	383
Burger King cheeseburger	350
Burger King chocolate shake	340
McDonald's Egg McMuffin	327
McDonald's Chicken McNuggets (without sauce)	314
McDonald's cheeseburger	307
Burger King hamburger	290
Burger King onion rings (regular)	270
McDonald's hamburger	255
Wendy's Hot Stuff Baked Potato (plain)	250
Wendy's chili	230
McDonald's french fries (regular)	220
Burger King french fries (regular)	210
Taco Bell Taco	186
Root beer (12 oz.)	155
Cola (12 oz.)	145
Kentucky Fried Chicken coleslaw	121
McDonald's Hash Browns	120
Coffee (black)	0

glasses and dishes; looking at other people's food; the breads, cheeses and crackers on the table. Then there is the menu, a kind of buffet on paper describing every item in detail and inviting the diner to try it all."

Still, the key to controlling your weight when dining out does not lie in the pastry cart or in the kitchen. It's you. By employing your own affirmative action plan—changing some habits, using a few tricks—you can easily learn to enjoy a great meal, feel satisfied and still be able to face the scale the next morning.

THE DINING EXPERIENCE— STEP BY STEP

The first step in dealing with eating out should actually come *before* you enter the restaurant. If at all possible, you should decide in advance what you're going to order. Dr. Musante suggests even writing it down, in an effort to keep you "honest." But you say you've never been to the restaurant before? No problem. Dr. Musante advises his patients simply to phone the establishment and inquire about the menu. You'll find most places quite willing to comply.

The key, explains Dr. Musante, is "to create as many controls as possible." When you arrive at the restaurant, and you have decided in advance to order, say, broiled trout, you avoid the temptation of seeing the menu and reading, possibly in fattening detail, about all the dishes you shouldn't be eating. "When it comes to ordering, the last thing you want to do is look at a menu," says Dr. Musante.

"Another helpful thing is to be the first one to order. What that does is a very interesting thing— we've found it sets the tone for the entire meal when people see what you order," he says.

At that point, the doctor says, the diner is practically "home free" by having turned the restaurant into a controllable setting.

If you can't avoid the menu, simply scan it, eyeballing only the sections you can regard as "safe," such as the "From the Broiler"

section or the poultry and fish selections. It's best to pretend the fried food section does not exist.

Another thing you might want to consider—especially if you must eat out a lot—is frequenting the same restaurant as much as possible. In addition to becoming familiar with the menu, Dr. Musante says, there's another thing that can work to the dieter's advantage: getting to know the waiters and waitresses, or even the chef. If they know the foods you favor and realize that you don't want your table cluttered with butter and rolls and other temptations, they will undoubtedly start to anticipate your requests.

Perhaps the most positive part of your eating-out plan is to recognize that you have plenty of options, during *every* phase of your meal.

Take the entree, for instance. If you have been a beef eater for years, there may be whole worlds you are missing at the restaurants you frequent. How about baked salmon, lean pork with bean sprouts or sauteed chicken breasts? Dr. Arnold Fox, the Beverly Hills, California, cardiologist and noted diet-book author, tells his patients to "look for fish or poultry on the menu. Ask for the fish broiled, without the sauce. Or just push the sauce away. Also, a lot of restaurants will make up a vegetable plate if you ask for one, but you won't find it on the menu." The idea is to be assertive— don't hesitate to ask for a dish prepared a special way.

That goes for side dishes, too. Don't hesitate to ask for a baked potato when french fries are posted as the choice of the day. When asked, "butter or sour cream?" answer, "a little yogurt" or "a sprinkling of herbs and pepper, please." And *always* ask how the vegetables are prepared. What may sound like a good deal calorically could turn out to be swimming in butter.

The same goes for the dinner salad. What can seem like a harmless addition can add up when you consider that most salad dressings come in at about 70 calories a tablespoon. Controlling your own portions is essential. So

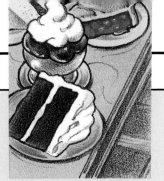

Beating the Dessert Trap

Row after row of chocolate cake, pies and pudding greet your eyes before you even get to the main dishes. It's no accident— it's a cafeteria line.

Often, the calorie-rich goodies are placed first in line, when you are hungriest and your will's the weakest. But there is a way to avoid it all. Join the line beyond the desserts so you don't even have to look at them. Or, if they're at the end of the line, as they *sometimes* are, breeze right by them (use the palm of your hand as a blinder if need be).

But dessert isn't the only pitfall in the cafeteria line that lures you to reach for more. Don't go for the multiple pats of butter and minicontainers of cream that are yours for the taking. One helping of each is more than enough.

get used to asking for the dressing on the side.

Another major roadblock comes when a waiter places a basket of rolls or bread in front of you. Most of the time, you automatically grab a piece, butter it and start chomping before you think about it. Yet, ask yourself: Are you eating the bread because it tastes so great and you are hungry, or because it will fill the time until your main course arrives? Keep in mind that one slice of bread is 60 to 70 calories, not counting the butter you spread on top—that's a lot of calories to occupy a few idle minutes! So, pass on it. Better yet, weight-control experts agree the best step is to just ask a waiter to remove the bread basket.

SAVE CALORIES: ORDER SIMPLE

No matter how often you eat out, keep one basic principle in mind: the simpler, the better. Stay away from casseroles or dishes bathed in sauces, because they are often laden with hundreds of calories.

Another good principle to follow that can help you get through the main course feeling lighter and unstuffed is to select a food that must be eaten slowly. Often, people—

What You Get When You Dine Out

U.S. STEAK HOUSE

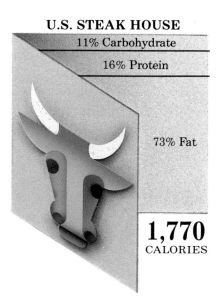

11% Carbohydrate

16% Protein

73% Fat

1,770 CALORIES

FRENCH

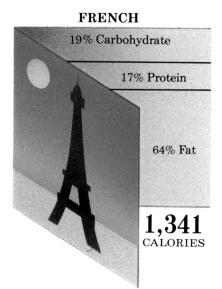

19% Carbohydrate

17% Protein

64% Fat

1,341 CALORIES

CHINESE

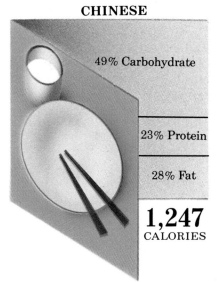

49% Carbohydrate

23% Protein

28% Fat

1,247 CALORIES

You're going out for dinner. Part of the reason, of course, is so you can experience some new and exciting tastes. So where will your taste buds take you—to French, Italian, Middle Eastern cuisines? And what will it all mean to your diet when you get there?

To find out, we called around to some of the most popular ethnic restaurants and asked what people ordered the most. Then, for specific recipes, we consulted our library of cookbooks and ran the recipes through a nutritionally programmed computer to discover what you might find in terms of calories, fat, protein and carbohydrates. As you can see below, the Mexican meal turned out to be

the kindest to your diet in terms of calories and fat, the Chinese and Italian were good in terms of fat. But the American steak house meal was the hardest on your diet in terms of calories *and* fat. Nevertheless, the steak house did have its strong point: In terms of cutting calories, it was the easiest to control. Here's what we tested.

U.S. Steak House. A 12-ounce sirloin steak (broiled), baked potato with sour cream, buttered broccoli and a salad with Russian dressing. While this meal is very high in calories and fat, you can do some cutting back by requesting yogurt instead of sour cream; lemon, not butter, on the broccoli;

particularly fidgety people—tend to keep nibbling (on rolls, their companion's side dishes or whatever's convenient) if they're the first ones finished. Imagine, however, how long you can savor crab legs (dipped in lemon, not butter sauce!) without doing damage weight-wise.

ORDERING SANDWICHES OUT

Sandwiches are among the foods that have suffered from a bad reputation for being "fattening." Most people who think sandwich think of the *bread* in terms of high calories. In most cases, however, it's what's *between* the bread that puts the sandwich on the forbidden list.

For starters, avoid luncheon meats and sandwich fillings made with mayonnaise and salad dressings, such as tuna, chicken and egg salads. Rather, go for sandwiches of lean meat or poultry. Always ask for whole grain bread. The fiber makes it more satisfying and fills you better. And take advantage of crunchy fillers such as lettuce, tomato, onion, sprouts and other vegetables. Also, search the menu for sandwiches that are open-faced. Cutting them takes extra time as you eat and you'll save the calories of that extra piece of bread.

MIDDLE EASTERN

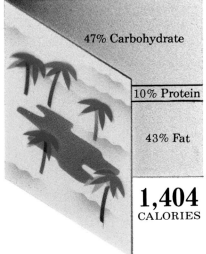

47% Carbohydrate

10% Protein

43% Fat

1,404
CALORIES

ITALIAN

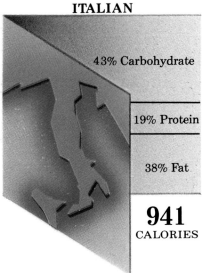

43% Carbohydrate

19% Protein

38% Fat

941
CALORIES

MEXICAN

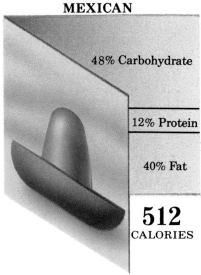

48% Carbohydrate

12% Protein

40% Fat

512
CALORIES

and wine vinegar on the salad. These substitutions alone can shave 350 calories and close to a third of the fat from the meal.

French. Chicken in cream sauce, crisp potato molds, peas braised in onions and salad with French dressing. The meal had the second highest fat content—64 percent.

Chinese. Chicken chow mein, wonton soup, a shrimp egg roll and white rice. While relatively low in fat, this meal turned out to be high in sodium.

Middle Eastern. Spinach-cheese pie, hummus with tahini (chick-peas), Arab bread, rice and salad with oil dressing. Of the 6 meals tested, this was the second highest in calories and the highest in sodium at 3,773 milligrams—over 18 times more than the 200 milligrams the average person needs each day.

Italian. Spaghetti with meat sauce, Italian bread and a salad with Italian dressing. This meal ran second best in two categories: calories and fat.

Mexican. Two tacos, a cup of gazpacho and rice. Not only was the meal lowest in calories, it also was lowest in sodium.

CROSSING THE 'I'M FINISHED' LINE

If you think of eating at a great restaurant and overcoming the temptations as the ultimate "competition" you'll face in losing weight, then you realize that the finish line is every bit as important as the starting line. The key is knowing when you've crossed it. Many of us were brought up with the idea that we should always finish what is on our plates. (Remember the starving children in China?) Social conscience aside, weight-control experts say the opposite—stop eating when you feel pleasantly satisfied, *not* stuffed— whether food is left or not. In fact, Dr. Musante tells his clients to "destroy" the leftovers on the plate by putting a lot of pepper or salt on them to avoid the temptation to nibble while others are eating. Better yet, get rid of your plate— fast. Give the waiter the cue that you are through by placing your fork, prongs up, diagonally across your plate.

DEALING WITH DESSERT

No tried-and-true weight watcher ever enters a restaurant with the intention of splurging on amaretto cheesecake or pecan pie. Often, however, we run into that well-meaning but thin-as-a-rail person who orders the sinfully delicious desserts and urges everyone else to "go ahead, treat yourself." So, go ahead—once in a while. Just because you're watching your weight doesn't mean you have to give up desserts forever.

But you can put a heavenly end to a meal without having to loosen your belt by ordering something

The Chef's Salad: A Pile of Calories

If the entree has the word "salad" in it, a lot of people see it as a green light to dig in, with little concern for calorie counting. But all that is green is not created equal. The popular chef's salad is the perfect example. It's about as good for your figure as a cheeseburger, french fries and a chocolate shake.

For all his good intentions, a chef packs a lot of calories on top of those greens. We asked one popular restaurant chef exactly what he puts on his salad and tallied up the calories. Here's what we came up with: 3 ounces of beef—186 calories; 3 ounces of turkey—134; 3 ounces of ham—155; 3 ounces of cheddar cheese—343; one hard-cooked egg—79; four ripe olives—26; a few slices of onion—5; lettuce—18; and half of a tomato—20 calories. The grand total: 966 calories. That's without the dressing, which often comes in a miniature urn, inviting you to pour it on. Considering that a single tablespoon of Italian, thousand island or blue cheese dressing is about 70 calories, your lunch can turn into a dieter's nightmare. Not only that, it's not all that good for you. A chef's salad is too high in fat and too low in fiber.

But if you are creative at home or a bit more assertive in restaurants, you can come up with a tasty alternative to a conventional chef's salad that's much lower in calories.

light, like berries in season or a fruit tart. And keep in mind that angel food cake is always a better choice than chocolate mousse, as is a cup of sherbet instead of ice cream pie. If you have an uncontrollable urge for something gooey, then share the treat with a friend.

Just keep in mind that dessert *is* a treat and it should stay that way. Make sure it remains the exception—never the rule. After all, you don't want to be wearing that chocolate cake long after the taste has worn away.

SHAVING FAST FOOD CALORIES

The fact that fast food establishments have had a huge impact on our diets is indisputable. Statistics show fast food sales amount to more than $19 billion per year, meaning that the average American spends $400 annually on eat-and-run fare. In 1982, Americans ate 376 percent more frozen potatoes, 78 percent more chicken and 17 percent more beef, and consumed 146 percent more soft drinks per capita than in 1962. Not coincidentally, these foods are major ingredients in fast food meals.

So, what are we getting for our fast food dollar? Ultimately, the fast food diner can pay a high price in calories for a minimum of nutrition, says Eleanor Young, Ph.D., a nutritionist at the University of Texas Health Science Center who, along with two dietitians, studied the nutritional content of foods at 11 chains. Take the double cheeseburger, french fries and dessert at one popular fast food chain. This typical fast food meal totals about 1,500 calories—almost the total minimum number of calories recommended for a young adult woman for an entire day (the average woman age 23 to 50

Here's our version of a "healthy chef's salad" that's a taste pleaser at only 318 calories per serving.

Makes 1 serving

  2 teaspoons olive oil
  1 teaspoon vinegar
 ⅛ clove garlic, minced
     pinch of ground cumin
     pinch of dried thyme
 ¼ teaspoon minced fresh parsley
2½ cups mixed salad greens
     (such as spinach, romaine
     and Chinese cabbage),
     lightly packed
 ⅓ cup cooked chick-peas
  2 tablespoons sliced mushrooms
  2 tablespoons cauliflower florets
  2 tablespoons broccoli florets
 ¼ red pepper, cut into julienne strips
 ½ hard-cooked egg, sliced
 ½ tomato, cut into small wedges
  3 thin slices red onion

To make the dressing, combine the oil, vinegar, garlic, cumin, thyme and parsley in a small bowl.

Place the salad greens in a large serving bowl. Add the chick-peas, mushrooms, cauliflower, broccoli and peppers. Toss with dressing. Arrange egg, tomato and onion on top.

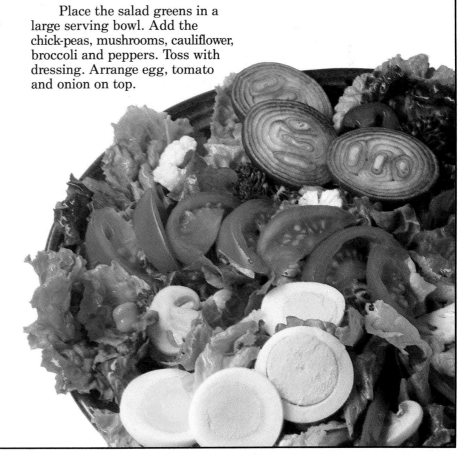

requires from 1,600 to 2,400 calories a day). Yet for all the calories, the meal doesn't even meet the U.S. Recommended Dietary Allowance for vitamins and minerals, the *minimum* nutrition we need to get through the day.

Worse for the dieter is the emphasis on "fast" in fast food. Such eat-and-run meals set the diner up to wolf down the food with lightninglike rapidity, before the stomach can signal the brain that it is stuffed to the seams. All too often, such meals leave the diner hungry and unsatisfied barely an hour later.

But vowing to stay out of a fast food restaurant—forever—is undoubtedly a promise few of us will ever keep. So you'll be happy to know there are ways to cut back on calories even at the fast food counter. The first thing to remember is that this is no place to be shy. Even though the food is often wrapped up and ready to go, the diet-conscious customer should realize that having it "your way" is the best way. At one chain, for example, if you ask for the ham and cheese sandwich without the sweet-and-sour mustard sauce, you will save yourself 50 calories. Hold the tartar sauce on the baked fish entree and you'll save 285 calories—more than the fish itself. Countless little steps will save you literally hundreds of calories. Get familiar with the calorie counts at your favorite fast food places (there are various calorie counters on the market that give such figures). By cutting a few calorie corners, the fast food line won't turn out to be the end of the line in your weight-control efforts—as long as you don't make getting in that line a habit.

BEWARE OF THE SALAD BAR

Perhaps one of the freshest options that has come along in a long while to aid the weight watcher is the salad bar. So common have they become in restaurants and fast food chains that there seems to be a little friendly competition as to who can lay out the best spread. At one chain, as many as 40 different fruits and vegetables are featured, including fresh watermelon and pineapple. Unfortunately, such a wide range of choices can get dieters into calorie trouble. Beyond the greens are such mayonnaise-laden goodies as potato salad, macaroni salad and coleslaw. There are beans or mushrooms swimming in oil, salami, ham or other meats for topping and enough varieties of cheese and salad dressing to put any diet program on red alert.

All this means that the only way to beat the salad bar is to stick with the items that are fresh and simple. It also helps to limit your trips to the salad bar to one. If the temptation of all the other choices is just too much, ask your waiter or

Overeating: An Occupational Hazard

Gael Greene knows all too well the challenge of facing an avalanche of chocolate truffles, berry tarts, juicy steaks, buttery sauces and crusty French bread day after day. As the nationally known restaurant critic for *New York* magazine, she has the delicious task of sampling the Big Apple's restaurants almost every night. She also has the awesome challenge of not letting the job literally go to her slim hips. How does she manage?

"First of all, I try never to finish everything, and since I eat out almost every night, I have no sense that this is my only chance," she says.

There are no foods she avoids, although she notes that she eats less meat than before. Rich, luscious desserts present the ultimate challenge. If she orders a chocolate dessert, for instance, she eats only a bite or two and then, "I quickly pass it to a friend."

At meals, Gael usually asks for water with a slice of lemon or lime; this helps her drink less wine.

But a critical part of her strategy—exercise—comes after the meal. "I exercise an hour a day, 6 days a week, and try to either dance after dinner or walk home, no matter where I am dining in the city . . . I have some friends who also love to walk, and sometimes we'll walk from Greenwich Village to 73rd Street."

Fine Dining on a Calorie Budget

Veal Escallope Parisienne served with Lentils in Tomato . . . White Wine Gelee with Kiwi Fruit . . . Grilled Swordfish with Pine Nuts. This is diet food? You bet it is. The Ambassador Grill, in New York City's plush United Nations Plaza Hotel, is among the growing number of establishments helping to prove that low-calorie food need not be low in enjoyment. The Ambassador Grill offers a 5-day-a-week rotating luncheon known as Menu Manhattan.

The meals, developed by the restaurant's chef and based on a special plan devised by the Mahoney Institute of the American Health Foundation, are all three courses—appetizer, entree and dessert—and add up to 550 calories or less. No more than 20 percent of the calories come from fat, a compromise between the more stringent 10 percent of some diet plans and the 30 percent recommended by the American Heart Association. A typical luncheon might include assorted vegetables with mustard sauce, grilled sole with orange, boiled potato, snow peas and cherry tomatoes and a dessert of a papaya with Grand Marnier liqueur. All that goodness adds up to only 450 calories—only 2 percent of which are from fat!

One meal you can find on the Ambassador Grill's Menu Manhattan is Melon with Air-Dried Beef, Broiled Salmon with Rice and Cherry Tomatoes, and Pear in Red Wine. It all comes to 406 calories and just 8.4 grams of fat.

"Our restaurant serves a big business crowd at lunchtime and we saw the need to offer this type of gourmet dining," says Robert M. Preissner, vice president of United Nations Development Corporation. Restaurant officials say the low-calorie meals have gone over well with Manhattan's midtown executives, who find the luncheons a refreshing change from the 3-martini, heavy midday meals of old. In his fast-paced business life, Preissner knows the dilemma often faced by executives who are watching their diets. "I watch my weight, but in a business like this, a lot is done over lunch and dinner," he says. "My technique has been to eat cheese, carrots and apples on the days I don't have to go out. Something like Menu Manhattan provides a nice alternative." So move over, cottage cheese. Here comes Menu Manhattan!

Tips for the Traveler

While traveling or on vacation, many people have a tendency to let their food intake veer upward faster than a jumbo jet. With a little preplanning and some self-control, you can take your taste buds on vacation without dreading getting reacquainted with the scale when you get home.

On the Plane

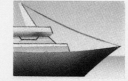

- Make arrangements with the airline in advance for a special low-cal dinner or lunch. Sometimes the preparation of these dishes is given more attention than the standard fare.
- Avoid drinking alcoholic beverages on board. Besides the obvious consequences, drinking can prompt fatigue, which could spark a binge later.
- Stick to your normal schedule of meals when crossing time zones. The fact that you experience 8 A.M. twice in one day is no excuse to eat two breakfasts.

On the Cruise Ship

- Eat only when you are hungry. So many meals are served on board it seems like you can find one almost every hour on the hour. Stick to 3 meals a day, just like at home.
- Take advantage of all fitness offerings on board, from classes in aerobic dance and slimnastics to deck games.
- Don't eat dessert at *every* meal. When you do, stick to those that feature fresh fruits.

In the Hotel

- Go European (no meals included), not American plan (meals prepaid). That way you won't feel obligated to eat a meal you otherwise could do without.
- Look for a hotel that has an exercise center or jogging trail. Visitors' centers and convention bureaus may be helpful in finding one.
- Unless you are staying in the penthouse (or close to it), avoid the elevators and walk the stairways. It's an easy way to burn calories.

In the Car

- Don't drive for hours on end without stopping for food. Studies have shown that alertness at the wheel begins to dwindle after about 1½ hours. And laboratory experiments indicate that food taken during a rest break restores driving abilities better than just a rest break alone. Pack a picnic lunch with wholesome and nourishing foods such as fresh fruit, dried fruit snack mixes and raw vegetables so you can control your diet destiny better.
- If you're traveling on the interstates, exit and go a few extra miles to find a place to eat. It's the best way to avoid the fast food areas.

waitress to get your salad for you and request salad greens, plenty of fresh vegetables and the dressing on the side. Or ask a friend to make the trip for you. Otherwise, you might do better ordering from the menu than going wild at the salad bar.

DRINKING—ADDING UP THE CALORIES

If you stood outside the window of many restaurants, you would notice a continuous motion among all the diners, much like the arms of a huge machine—the frequent lifting of glasses. Probably then, too, you would realize just how many people there are who feel eating and drinking go hand in hand.

Think of it—the three-martini lunches, beer and pizza, before-dinner cocktails, after-dinner liqueurs, wine- and cheese-tasting parties. Such drinking habits add 62,000 calories per year to the average American's diet.

If you want to think of the cumulative effect of even a little bit of drinking, take the hypothetical woman who sticks to diet soda at lunch but likes to enjoy her dinner with two glasses of white wine. At 80 calories for each 3½-ounce glass, she consumes an extra 1,120 calories per week, or more than 58,000 calories a year! That amount is enough to create and maintain about 12 pounds of fat. So drinking is indeed a part of eating out that can make a big difference weight-wise.

Since drinking alcoholic beverages often is a ritual in dining out, the same plan-ahead strategy that weight-control experts advise for controlling food applies to alcohol. If you know, for instance, that you must go out for a business lunch tomorrow, decide ahead of time to order just one weak drink—perhaps a wine spritzer—even if you're sure your colleagues will be sipping martinis. Drinking a little, or even not drinking at all, is perfectly acceptable, even in business or social circles. "If drinks are being offered, it's socially acceptable to order soda water or mineral water," says John D. Adams, Ph.D., a lifestyle-management expert from

Arlington, Virginia. "And this goes for someone who is entertaining a client. Attitudes have changed. Years back, if I ordered mineral water I'd get a hard time from the people I was with for not drinking. Now it's quite natural to avoid alcohol at lunch, even in Washington where the multimartini lunch is still a very real thing."

If you feel you want to join an associate or friend in a cocktail, order drinks that are light in calories. A spritzer, a combination of white wine and club soda, can go a long way if you go heavy on the soda water. In fact, some folks even ask for soda water with a splash of wine and a twist of lemon. Served in a tall glass, this drink can be sipped slowly and can help your diet escape many a social occasion unscathed. Or simply order mineral water.

If your favorite drink is hard liquor, keep in mind that the higher the proof, the greater the calories. One and one-half ounces of 90-proof liquor has 110 calories, while the same amount of 100-proof has 15 calories more. Add the calories of mixers like ginger ale or tonic, and you get a good idea how "hard" hard liquor will be on your weight.

EATING ON THE ROAD

Breakfast, lunch and dinner on the road can often wreak havoc on a weight-control regimen. A harrying schedule can make us eat too fast. Being among good fun and good friends can make us eat too much. And the dull spots we encounter during *any* trip can make us eat too often—just to break the boredom.

Whether we're traveling for business or pleasure, eating on the road requires extra effort.

Finding a place that meets your personal desires needn't happen just by chance. Plan ahead by perusing books and guides or writing to the visitors' bureau of the town you'll be visiting for restaurant information.

Expert travelers have their own strategies. Physical fitness expert and TV personality Jack LaLanne, for example, says he chooses places by "instinct" by looking for cleanliness and other signs. Wherever he

travels, LaLanne makes special requests for certain foods just as if he was lunching near home.

"I'll call the maitre d' over and tell him I want my salad prepared a certain way. I'll even bring my own seasonings like garlic and onion powders. If the guy is a little contrary, I'll buy him a bottle of wine or I'll tip him. I'll do anything to get what I want," says LaLanne.

LaLanne recommends that those traveling on a limited budget seek out the best cafeteria in town: "You have a multiple choice right there with foods like broiled or baked fish, salads, vegetables and fruit juices."

You can also look for natural foods or vegetarian restaurants in the telephone book or call the manager of a health food store to ask for names of restaurants that offer healthy food. You may also want to call a local health spa in the area where you are staying and ask for a recommendation for a good place to eat well and stay thin. Many restaurants within hotels also may have special meals not even listed on the menu, or may make up a special dieter's delight, if asked.

None of these approaches means you have to suffer. In fact, it can be a rewarding challenge to determine what the local specialties are and how they can fit into your weight-loss plan. An island vacation, for instance, can mean great *and* calorie-economic local delicacies like conch and dolphin. Be mindful of how they are prepared, though, since this could mean extra calories. Or you can feast on locally grown produce.

All in all, there's no reason for you to avoid a certain restaurant's specialty and later feel regretful. Treat yourself, but wisely. No one should have to deprive himself of some of the best clam chowder in existence if vacationing on the coast of Maine or of great pancakes bursting with blueberries at some roadside stop in the South. Just be sure to keep these tips in mind: Make sure that you are hungry before you eat, eat slowly and stop when you feel *pleasantly* satisfied. What you see in the mirror when you arrive home will be the thanks for your efforts.

5

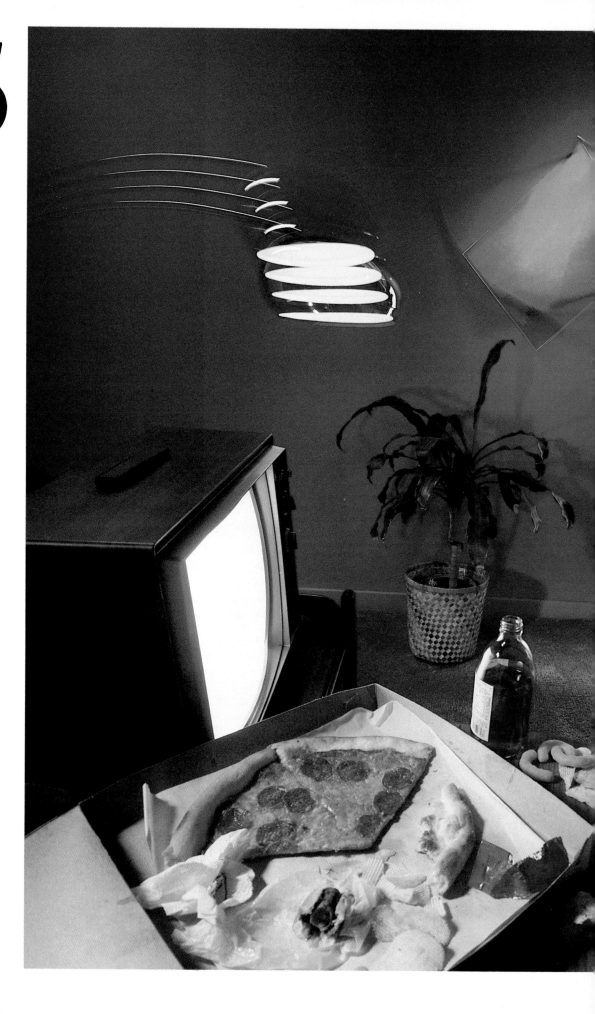

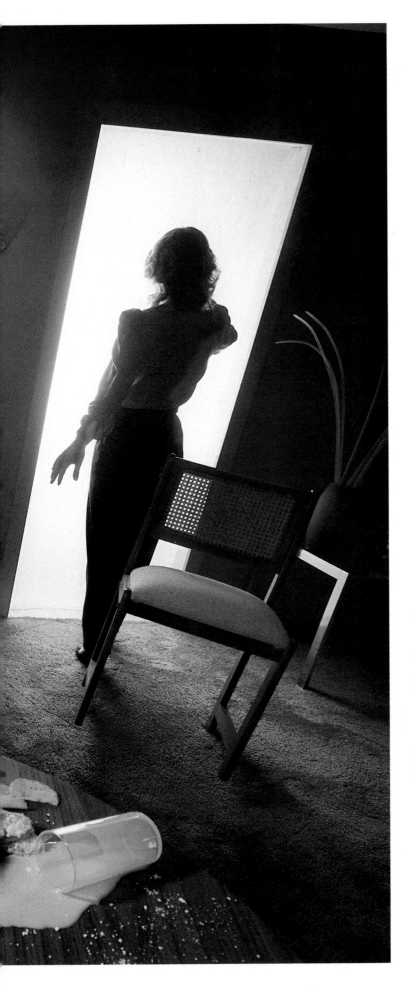

Eating—Out of Control

Do you get the urge to binge?
Find out why—and how
you can stop it.

Do you ever have a day like this one? The sign catches your eye on the drive home from Saturday grocery shopping: "Fastest and Tastiest Tex-Mex in Town." You decide on an impulse that you want a burrito and the shopping bags in the back seat jostle as you turn sharply into the parking lot of the fast food restaurant. A bag of chocolate chip cookies rips as it falls to the seat, scattering the cookies. Muttering to yourself, you pick up two cookies. They're just crumbs on your lips by the time you enter the restaurant and order a quick burrito and a side order of guacamole. You wolf down the "snack" and take the complimentary tortilla chips with you for the drive home. The sound of pop music on the car radio is almost drowned out by the crunch you make chewing on the chips you mindlessly plop into your mouth. You don't feel full or satisfied or even hungry, just driven by an overwhelming urge to eat.

The rest of the family is out of the house until evening, leaving you free from anyone's watchful eye. As you put several cans in the cupboard, you pick at a few of the cookies from the open bag. You find a little peanut butter left in the old jar and spread it on some saltines; no sense leaving the old jar around when there's a new jar just waiting to be opened. One bag of groceries is unpacked and put safely away. You start working on the other bags. A package of bite-size candy bars is put in its hiding place, but only after you take out three of them and toss them into your mouth. You put the vegetables in their bin and the milk, mayonnaise and pickles in their spot inside the refrigerator door—all but two of the pickles, that is. You eat them. You've finally put everything away except some barbecued chicken from the grocery store deli, a large bag of potato chips and green onion dip.

Although you're not really hungry after eating the Mexican food, peanut butter crackers, pickles, cookies and candy bars, you stuff yourself with this "lunch" until your stomach hurts.

You're on a binge, an eating jag, a pig-out. And you're not alone. Binging is something a lot of us have in common.

AS AMERICAN AS THREE SLICES OF APPLE PIE

Binging, in fact, is as much a part of the American lifestyle as baseball or Sunday afternoon drives. Ask any of your friends if they have ever binged and, if they're honest, most will answer yes.

"Probably everyone will binge at some time in their life," says Phyllis Fleming, Ph.D., associate director of the public health nutrition program at the University of Minnesota in Minneapolis. "If you do binge, don't feel guilty—guilt is destructive. Binging can be okay once in a while. If you do it just for the joy of eating, there is nothing to feel guilty about."

After all, sometimes we're actually *encouraged* to binge. Take American holidays like Thanksgiving and the Fourth of July—a whole day off from work to feast and picnic with family and friends. What could be wrong with that? Nothing, of course. Holiday feasting is fun and basically harmless. A return to normal eating the following day will usually put the body back on a healthy track.

Unfortunately, not all binges are so innocent, carefree and infrequent. For some people, binging becomes a habit. A dangerous, fat-building habit. As Dr. Fleming says, an occasional binge isn't harmful "just as long as it isn't hurting you physically and you aren't using it as a crutch or coping method. The time to worry is when food is used to fix problems. It never will." In fact, it can quickly make them worse. One study even goes so far as to suggest that you are a binge eater if you eat for emotional reasons as few as three times a month.

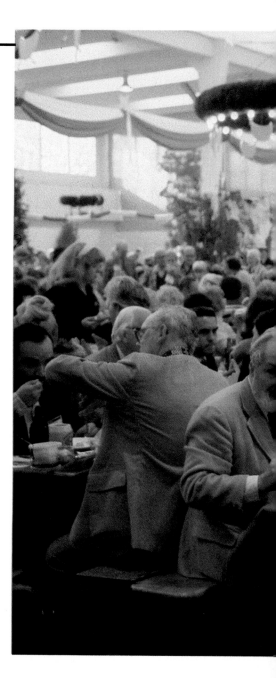

BINGING: A VICIOUS CYCLE

There are plenty of problems associated with an appetite that's out of control. The first one is obvious: You'll start to gain weight. Eventually, a more severe problem will arise: the vicious cycle of binging and dieting.

Most people feel good while they overeat. It satisfies something deep within. But guilt and depression are the usual post-binge emotions. Because we don't feel good about ourselves, we binge again. The vicious cycle is set in motion.

But binging doesn't only play games with our minds. It isn't good for our bodies, either. Overeating

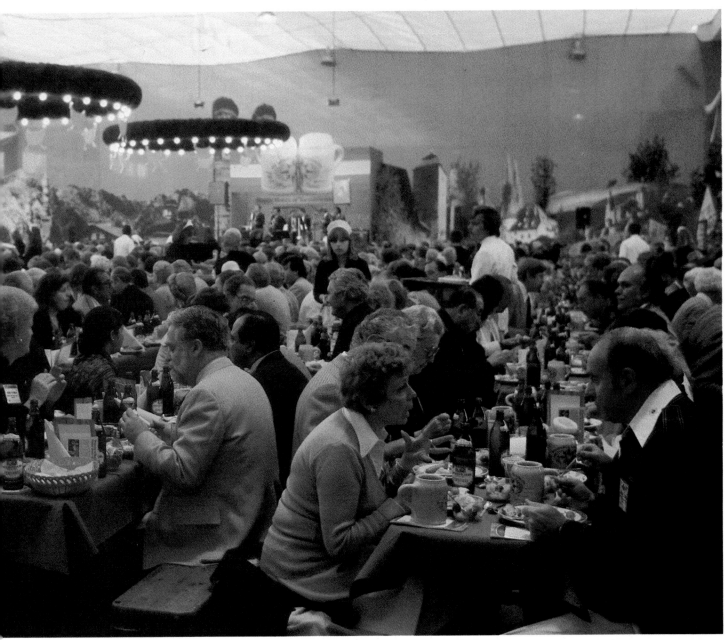

puts a real burden on the body. Overloading the system with food puts a tremendous strain on the stomach, causing the body to divert extra blood to the digestive tract. It can also make you tired and listless. Overdoing it before bedtime can cause heartburn, poor sleep and impotence. Some people have even attributed their migraines and arthritis to binging.

Like any bad habit, the binge cycle can be broken. There are ways to remain binge free forever. The first step is understanding why you binge. Unfortunately, there is no simple answer. Binging often involves a complex mix of emotional and physical factors. Let's examine some of the common and not-so-common ones and see if there's an answer that may work for you.

UNDEREATING LEADS TO OVEREATING

One truth about the human appetite is that it doesn't take kindly to being put on hold. Frustrate your taste buds and they'll frustrate you. A psychologist from the University of London found after studying the eating habits of 68 medical students that dietary denial leads to dietary excess. The researcher discovered that the greatest abstainers were also the greatest binge eaters, *and* the most overweight.

There's a definite moral in this
(continued on page 80)

Plenty of food, plenty of drink, plenty of laughs. There are times when out-and-out overindulgence is expected—even sanctioned. After all, people come from all over the world to do just that at Munich, Germany's annual Oktoberfest. Some 10 million revelers drop in each year for the 16-day eating and drinking feast. Some estimates put total consumption at 4 million quarts of beer, 1 million sausages, 50 tons of fish, nearly half a million chickens and countless numbers of roast oxen.

Are You a Foodaholic?

This test will help you examine your eating habits to see if you are a destructive eater—a foodaholic. Taking the test will help you become aware of when and why you binge. Apply the questions to your own situation and be honest. Rate your answers on a scale of 4 to 0 like this: 4=usually; 3=frequently; 2=sometimes; 1=rarely; 0=never. An analysis of the totals follows the test.

Foodaholism: The Food Fixation
1. Are you preoccupied with food and your next opportunity to eat?
2. Have you missed what someone was saying because you were thinking about food?
3. At parties, is the buffet like a magnet to you?
4. Have you made mistakes at work because you were thinking of food?
5. Does staying in touch with food make it hard for people to get in touch with you? *Example:* Because of your trips to the office candy machine, you are missing important phone calls.
6. Have you encountered a potentially dangerous situation while driving because your attention was on eating?

The Food-Centered Lifestyle
1. Is what to serve your first decision when planning a party?
2. Do you have friends who are *primarily* eating or dieting buddies?
3. Is eating out your chief form of entertainment?
4. Do your conversations focus on food, restaurants, recipes or diets?
5. Are you disappointed when your companions are reluctant to go to your favorite restaurant?
6. Do you select and anticipate even before you arrive what you'll be eating at home, at a party or at a restaurant even when you've eaten within four hours and are not genuinely hungry?

The Fast Foodaholic
1. Do you eat quickly?
2. Do you wonder where your food went, because you do not remember finishing it?
3. Are you through eating before everyone else?
4. Do you eat your food without tasting it very much?
5. Do you find you've barely enjoyed your meal, snack or binge?

The Closet Foodaholic
1. Do you have some preference for eating alone?
2. Would you prefer not having others see what, how much or how often you eat?
3. Do you eat sparingly with others, and consume more later?
4. Do you snack behind the scenes while you are helping, visiting, or preparing foods?
5. Do you eat in your car?

The Food Fix-up
1. Do you use food as medicine?
2. Do you seek food when you have a problem to solve?
3. Do you have specific foods or quantities of food which you use to help you handle uncomfortable emotions? *Example:* Eating a hot fudge sundae for lunch when you feel nervous about an important afternoon meeting.

4. Do you use food to fill the void inside you or in your life? *Example:* Preparing cinnamon toast and hot chocolate, just like Mom did, on a Saturday night when you wish you were out on a date.
5. Do you eat to relieve tiredness or boredom or to keep yourself awake?
6. Do you eat to help you sleep?
7. Do you eat when you're not hungry, because you *might get hungry* if you don't?

The Snack Thief
1. Do you hide food or sneak it?
2. Have you lied about what or how much you've eaten?
3. Have you stolen food or money to buy it in order to support your habit?
4. Are you stingy or ungenerous with your food supply?
5. Do you feel strong emotion toward someone who tampers with your food supply?

The Forced Feeder
1. Do you feel powerless over food?
2. Do you eat more than you planned?
3. Do you eat even when you're not hungry?
4. Do you eat foods you do not especially like?
5. Do other people determine what you will eat? *Examples:* Eating to please the host who keeps filling your plate; rewarding Grandma for making what she thinks is your favorite food by enthusiastically gobbling it and asking for more, even though you are actually not too fond of it.

Feast or Famine
1. How frequently are you engaged in either an eating binge or an attempt to diet?

Foodaholic Defenses

Denial
How Often Do You Tell Yourself . . .
1. Sure, I eat destructively. Doesn't everybody?
2. Sure, I live on junk food, but I'm not fat.
3. Lots of people eat more than I do.
4. My gorging didn't make me feel this awful. It's lack of sleep.
5. I skipped lunch (while eating 3,000 calories to make up for it).
6. A little bit won't hurt (as you start on your favorite binge food).
7. I ate very little today (not counting snacks).

Delusions
1. Other people tell me I'm much fatter/thinner than I think I am.
2. I used to be fat/thin, and I still picture myself that way.
3. I'm amazed at how fat/thin I look in photographs.

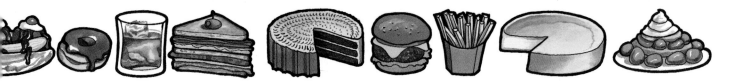

Rigidity

1. I think my problems would be solved if I could just get organized, but other people insist I'm already overorganized.
2. I'm compulsively neat.
3. I have specific times for given activities, and I feel unnerved by deviations from my schedule.
4. I exercise rigorously and regularly, and when I can't, I feel very anxious.
5. Sitting still and relaxing is distressing for me.
6. If I do something wrong, I worry that everyone will think less of me.
7. There just aren't enough hours in the day for all I have to do.

Blaming

Do You Tell Yourself or Others . . .

1. We live in a food-oriented society; my eating is normal among my group.
2. Those tempting foods on TV are part of the problem.
3. The hostess will be hurt if I don't eat her food.
4. I have to have all that junk food around for my teenagers.
5. My spouse is skinny and needs fattening foods.
6. My customers expect large, elaborate meals when I take them out.

Rationalization

How Often Do You Think . . .

1. Oh, well, it's a vacation.
2. My family runs to fat, anyway.
3. I think it's my metabolism.
4. I haven't had pie for ages, so 2 pieces tonight is okay.
5. After all, I've gotten rid of all my other vices. I have to have some fun in life.

Self-Ridicule

Do You Say or Think . . .

1. I'm just a jolly, fat person.
2. Here comes the garbage disposal—me!
3. I'd be just the right weight if I were 6 inches taller.
4. You don't have to worry about leftovers when I'm around.
5. I'm not allowed to have second helpings. So I'll just skip them and go right to thirds.

Intellectualizing

How Often Do You Tell Yourself or Others . . .

1. People in our family have a tendency to eat as a conflict-avoidance mechanism.
2. Our culture is chemophilic, fondly believing that there is a substance to cure any problem.
3. The media and manufacturers establish the norms in our society by creating a demand for specific food products.

The Foodaholic's Best Friend

How often have these statements or similar ones been directed to you?

1. We're on vacation. I want to see the sights, not only the restaurants.
2. Don't eat now. There's a big meal coming.
3. A third helping? Where do you put it all?
4. How can you still be hungry? That meal was huge.
5. I was saving that piece of cake for Mitzi.
6. All we do is go out and eat. I want to do something different this weekend.
7. Your crunching all during the movie bothered me.
8. Yes, it's time for lunch, but we should complete our agenda before we break.
9. I know the food at Le Gourmet is great, but we'll be late for the movie if we go there.
10. I'm so glad you picked up the prescription for Belinda's earache. Oh, I see you got a pizza, too. What, you forgot the prescription?
11. Yes, that dinner-theater serves good food, but they have rotten plays. What's more important, the food or the play?
12. It's true, this airline is notorious for its crummy cuisine. But I have never seen anyone get so thoroughly upset over a bad meal.
13. We keep talking about food, recipes, restaurants. Tell me, have you read any good books lately?

Foodaholism Total

Below 115. You aren't a foodaholic, although you may have occasional bouts of less-than-healthy eating. Your real problem may be how unforgiving you are of yourself for that behavior.

115-130. You have a tendency toward foodaholism. Review your test scores and note if there is one specific area in which you score relatively high, or have a cluster of 3's or 4's. If this is your scoring pattern, you could be a single-issue foodaholic. It is also possible that you are less than 15 percent overweight, and keep inflicting a diet on yourself and then rebelling. You might stop abusing food if you stopped scolding yourself and simply allowed yourself to eat healthy foods and quantities. Perhaps you are a person who was reared with constant comments about what you did or did not eat, and now you are continuing the same running commentary in your head. Were you to send this resident critic in your head on a Hawaiian vacation, your preoccupation with food might diminish noticeably.

130-170. You are a full-scale foodaholic. Remember, you probably did not develop your destructive eating patterns overnight. Do not be impatient or unfair to yourself by expecting an immediate recovery and lifestyle change.

From *The Food Fix*, by Sandra Gordon Stoltz. ©1983 by Prentice-Hall, Inc. Reprinted by permission of Prentice-Hall, Inc.

Excuses, Excuses

Placing blame doesn't make binging any better. Avoid using these common excuses:

• "Since I already blew my diet by eating a pizza at lunch, I might as well keep enjoying myself."

• "I'm going to quit eating sweets tomorrow, so I might as well go whole hog today."

• "There's no sense wasting food, so I might as well finish the rest of the lasagna."

• "I'm under a work deadline and just can't be bothered with watching what I eat."

• "It doesn't matter how much I eat this weekend because I'm going on a diet Monday."

• "There's nothing else to do; at least I can eat."

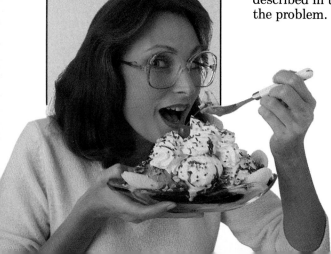

study for the chronic dieter. Severe dieting can be self-defeating.

Low-calorie diets of, say, 1,200 calories a day or less may help you shed pounds—if you can stick with them. Unfortunately, most people shed their diets more quickly than they shed pounds. "The biggest reason people start to binge is because they starve themselves, and it is very demoralizing to fail this way after sticking to a restricted diet," says Dr. Arnold Andersen of the Johns Hopkins University Eating and Weight Disorders Clinic in Baltimore. This type of dieting is often called restrained eating because the dieter is making a serious, conscious effort to control his eating.

"By consciously, we mean they are counting calories and they're skipping dessert because they know they can't have it," says Dr. Thomas Wadden, of the University of Pennsylvania. "These people tend to eat when they are depressed or upset. And depression and being upset prevent them from exercising their control. It's saying, 'Well, geez, I'm just too wiped out from being too upset about the things at work to worry about food right now.'" These people might comfort themselves by eating "just one" candy bar. As soon as they eat one, they figure they've completely blown their diet anyway, so they go on a binge. "They feel it's a total loss already," says Dr. Wadden. The vicious cycle appears again.

One way to be less vulnerable to these attacks is to give up crash dieting. Don't restrict your diet to the point where you have cravings in the first place. A well-balanced eating plan that includes a variety of natural foods—like the plan described in this book—should solve the problem.

THE EMOTIONAL OUTLET

After a bad day at work, do you ever come home and stuff yourself with an entire box of cookies? Does a fight with your spouse precipitate an uncontrollable urge to eat everything in sight? Do you "pig out" on junk food after a poor night's sleep? If you answer yes to any one of these, your mood swings may be the cause of your eating problems.

Dr. Wadden doesn't think it's necessary to give in to these mood swings. He first has his patients make a record of when they binge and what mood sets off the eating jag. A binger must ascertain why he binges. Dr. Wadden asks, "What are the circumstances under which you binge? You don't have a date Friday night? You got a lousy grade on an exam? Identify those high-risk situations before they come up and plan to do something else instead of binge at those times." There *are* alternatives to binging, and they'll make you feel better in the long run.

"Binging caused by tension, fatigue and boredom isn't a healthy outlet at all," says Dr. Fleming. "Binging is an unhealthy way to take care of your problems. It's like smoking and drinking. There are better ways."

Dr. Fleming tells her clients to assess their binging behavior first, and then make changes in their environment and habits so they can avoid the binge triggers. "Modify the factors that start a binge," says Dr. Fleming. "If you are bored, go for a walk. If you are angry, yell your head off. If you're tired, lie down for ten minutes. You'll find that these things will squelch your desire to binge."

If the urge to eat is so overwhelming that you feel you just can't quell it, then go ahead and eat. Just pay attention to what you are doing. If you are in the habit of binging on a loaf of bread while making dinner after work, try taking only one piece of bread out of the bag and putting the rest away. Don't leave the loaf on the counter where it will tempt you. Put it in the freezer, if you must. Dr. Fleming

Chocolate—The Sinful Snack

Some people like to drink in public, smoke in public and occasionally even swear in public. But only in their own company do some people dare indulge in their most secret passion: munching on fistfuls of chocolate candy.

Strange? Perhaps. But far from unusual. To some extent, nearly all of us are locked in an intense and ridiculous love-hate relationship with this unique confection.

So, what is it that makes chocolate so irresistible? Philip G. Keeney, Ph.D., a professor of food sciences at Pennsylvania State University, believes he has the answer. "Guilt," he says matter-of-factly. "We're always on the defensive because we don't eat it for nutrition. The wages of sin make it taste that much better."

Indeed, chocolate seems to be the perennial scapegoat that physicians, dietitians and even rabid connoisseurs hate to love. Perhaps with good reason. During the last several decades, scientific literature has pointed to chocolate for its alleged role in such maladies as migraines, acne, dental cavities and heartburn. And, at a delicious 150 calories per ounce, it has a sneaky tendency to make us fat.

But people go on craving it anyway. In fact, some people's desire for chocolate seems almost as if they were possessed. What's behind their behavior? "If you eat chocolate to feel better, be more energetic and alert or for a sense of well-being, it suggests an addiction." says Marshall Mandell, M.D.

Although no doctor, psychologist or nutritionist interviewed recommended an outright ban on chocolate, the consensus is that overconsumption invites abuse. The collective catchword is "moderation."

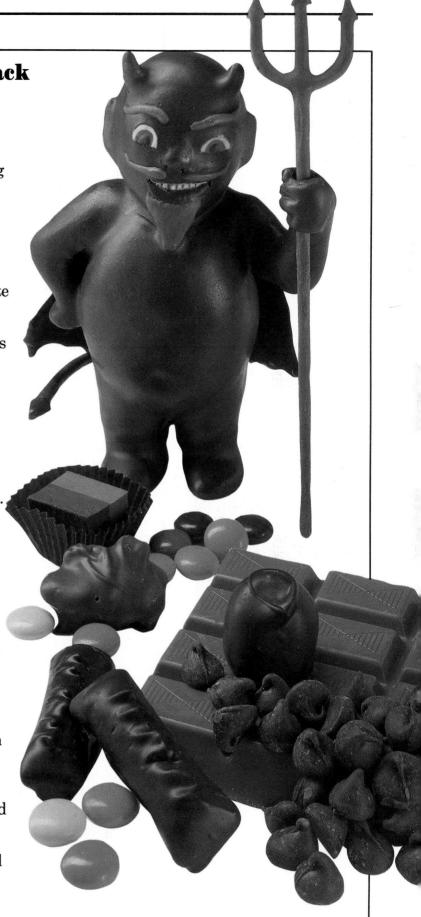

Don't Let Sugar Sneak Up on You

Chances are there's a lot of sugar hiding on your pantry shelves. It can show up in the most unlikely products. So, be sure to scan food labels before you buy (the ingredients are listed in descending order by amount). Some examples of "hidden sugar products" and their percentages are:

- Nondairy creamer, 56.9%.
- Russian dressing, 30.2%.
- Ketchup, 28.9%.
- French dressing, 23%.
- Canned peaches, 17.9%.
- Blueberry yogurt, 13.7%.
- Bouillon cubes, 14.8%.
- Crackers, 12%.
- Canned corn, 10.7%.
- Peanut butter, 9.2%.
- Spaghetti sauce, 6.2%.

Also, many breakfast cereals contain a lot of sugar. Fight back by reading labels.

also recommends keeping fresh, washed vegetables handy in the refrigerator. "If you absolutely must, you can eat the whole bag if you want. You'll feel better physically, and won't feel so guilty," she says. In extreme cases, Dr. Fleming tells people to actually hide the offending food. "Some people even put it so high and far away that they have to get a ladder to reach it," she says.

If these steps don't cure your binging, you might be the victim of a more physical dependence. Scientific research has shown that certain foods can actually trigger a binge. Some people aren't stretching the truth when they say eating makes them hungry.

"The main foods people become dependent on are flour, refined carbohydrates (which quickly turn to sugar in the body) and sugar," says Mehl McDowell, M.D., an associate clinical professor of psychiatry at the University of California at Los Angeles. "Sugar is the most common."

THE SUGAR ROLLER COASTER: A DANGEROUS RIDE

Sugar is a major factor in the vicious up-and-down cycle that a lot of binge eaters are on. People who binge on sugar are like cigarette addicts. The sugar satisfies their immediate craving, but the satisfaction is short-lived and the cravings start again. Through a series of chemical changes in the body, sugar sets up the binger for failure.

According to Dr. McDowell, anyone can turn into a sugar addict. The reason sugar is so addictive is because it plays games with the body's insulin and blood sugar levels. Glucose, another name for blood sugar, is what keeps our bodies going. It's like coal for a furnace. If the blood sugar gets too low or too high, our bodies don't work up to par. A gland called the pancreas produces the insulin that regulates the amount of blood sugar in the body. When you eat sugar, especially the quickly absorbed refined sugars, blood sugar goes up. Then, the pancreas releases insulin to balance the blood sugar level.

Unfortunately, the insulin is so overeffective that it causes the blood sugar levels to drop too far below normal before they balance out. This drop in blood sugar levels causes a craving for more sugar. It's like a roller coaster that refuses to stop.

Some people overcompensate for this drop in blood sugar by binging. Maybe they'll eat a dozen cookies instead of one or two, or drink three colas instead of their usual cup of tea. The binge will make them feel better, but only for a short while. The truth is that they are just setting themselves up for another failure, another binge. The sweets they eat to raise their sugar levels will just cause the pancreas to release another onslaught of insulin, repeating the whole process. It is an ongoing cycle, a catch-22.

Recall your binges. Do you binge primarily on sugary or refined carbohydrate foods? If so, sugar may be the culprit. The best way to test whether or not you are a sugar addict is to see what happens when you give up sugar and refined carbohydrates completely and suddenly. If, after a day or two, you feel cranky, exhausted, confused or shaky and have a strong craving for sugar, you've got a sugar "addiction."

One survey showed that 37 percent of the average American's diet is composed of sugary foods, desserts, beverages, condiments, fats and oils. Sugar consumption is clearly a major problem. But it is a problem that can be overcome. Unlike protein, water and vitamin C, sugar is one thing we can live without. As John Yudkin, M.D., writes in *Sweet and Dangerous*, ". . . there is no physiological requirement for sugar; all human nutritional needs can be met in full without having to take a single spoon of white or brown or raw sugar, on its own or in any food or drink."

Just how does a person with a sweet tooth give up sugar? One way is to go cold turkey. But for some people, that's hard, if not impossible, to do. Another strategy is to make yourself aware of just how much sugar you are eating, and cut back on it. Read food labels. You'll be surprised at the amount of "hidden" sugar in many of your favorite foods. Many canned soups have sugar. So do ketchup, mayonnaise, tomato sauce and flavored yogurt. Sugar also goes by different names. Turbinado, sucrose, glucose, fructose, galactose, dextrose, levulose, lactose, maltose, corn syrup, corn sugar, maple syrup, honey, sorbitol, mannitol and hexitol are all common forms of sugar.

Another tip: Banish all sugar from the house. It makes it much more difficult to feed the sugar urge when it arises. Nibble on good snack foods—vegetables, fruits, nuts or cheese. Staying satisfied throughout the day helps keep cravings under control.

Certain vitamins and minerals also help assuage a sugar craving. The B vitamins play an important role because they help keep blood sugar at an optimum level. The mineral chromium helps insulin do its job efficiently. And zinc and manganese help stabilize blood sugar, particularly when it's at an ebb. But zinc has an added benefit. It helps enhance taste acuity. One study found that when people increased their zinc levels, their taste buds became more acute, particularly when it came to sugar. The sweet taste of sugar became almost too sweet.

Exercise is another way to forget about sugar. "If you want sugar, get down on the floor and do a couple of push-ups," says Ray Wunderlich, M.D., of St. Petersburg, Florida. "It'll put you in a whole new frame of mind."

FOOD ALLERGIES: ANOTHER CAUSE OF OVEREATING

If cutting back on sugar doesn't keep you from binging, your problems might be due to a bad reaction to some other food. Many doctors now believe that people can actually develop allergies to any food—and that the allergies can manifest as anxiety, depression or a host of other emotional snake pits. To make matters worse, the food that triggers the allergy—the bad feeling—can also temporarily get rid of it if you eat *large* amounts of that food. And

Binging in the Danger Zone

While common, occasional binging can usually be overcome with a little effort and dietary changes, there is another type of binging that is far more serious. Bulimia is the name of this binge disease, and it is believed to affect almost 1 in 5 college-age women. The afflicted are obsessed with food and will go to great lengths to ingest huge numbers of calories—up to 20,000 a day in some cases—and then, stuffed to the point of physical discomfort and psychologically disturbed by how much they have eaten, they will seek to purge the food from their bodies with laxatives or by vomiting.

This purging keeps bulimics from gaining weight. Unlike those who suffer from a closely related disease, anorexia nervosa, bulimics don't necessarily become emaciated, because, aside from the binges, they usually eat a normal, healthy diet. However, this doesn't mean that they don't have any problems. The physical strain of vomiting can cause tears in the lining of the esophagus, depletion of vitamins and minerals and a host of other problems. Laxatives can become addictive after prolonged use, a dependency that results from recurring constipation. The disease is also psychologically devastating, causing tremendous guilt and self-doubt.

Bulimia has been attributed to many causes, ranging from a reaction to certain foods to emotional stress. No one knows for sure what causes the disease. What is certain, however, is that if you are gorging and then purging yourself with any regularity, you should seek help from a physician or therapist. Bulimia is a complex disease—too complex to tackle on your own.

there's even another monkeywrench— the allergy is hidden, so that most people fail to link the food to the onrush of negative feeling. So you eat a food, you get in a bad mood and your body automatically craves more of that food so you can feel good again. The exact mechanism of this food/mood allergy is unknown, but the end result is a cycle of eating and craving that is very similar to sugar addiction.

Dr. McDowell became curious about food allergies following a personal bout with binging and overweight. In 1968 he was lugging an extra 30 pounds around when he

Seeing red and feeling blue—you know what these phrases mean. But did you know that colors actually influence your mood? Restaurant designers often devise color schemes that will prompt people to eat and encourage a fast turnover at tables. Red, orange and yellow are popular with many fast food chains, probably because they are "hot," stimulating colors. These colors also are effective in road signs—they seem to draw you off the highway and into the restaurant. So, the next time your appetite suddenly perks up when you enter a fast food place, take a minute to look around. The colors that drew you in to the restaurant may also cause you to order more food than you really want.

got fed up with being heavy. "That was a lot of weight to carry around on my short frame," recalls Dr. McDowell, "but I lost it. And I've kept it off since."

What's his secret? An old Chinese custom. Dr. McDowell had been searching in vain for a simple rule that would help him and his patients lose weight and keep them from binging. He got into a discussion with a friend who had traveled in China who marveled at how lean most Chinese people are. McDowell asked him the secret and he replied that the Chinese diet included only small amounts of processed flour and sugar. McDowell thought about the Chinese diet and coined the simple rule: Don't eat glue foods.

Glue foods are anything containing refined carbohydrates—sugar and flour. "These are the most common addictive foods," says McDowell. "People always seem to binge on carbohydrates, or, more rarely, fruits. You don't often find people binging on brown rice or fresh vegetables."

The rule is simple: Give up cakes, sugar, white bread and most types of junk foods. But giving up these foods is not very easy for most people who are addicted to them. McDowell teaches his patients a

behavior technique to get them over their cravings. "If a patient has a desire for a dish of chocolate ice cream, for instance, I instruct him to immediately picture that ice cream 'glued' into disgusting fat deposits on his abdomen. With sufficient repetition of such imaginary scenes, this 'disgust' feeling becomes associated with that type of food in real-life encounters. The patient is further instructed to deliberately and instantly, throughout his waking life, react to every real-life reminder of his enemy foods with this strong, vivid disgust response. He then immediately rewards himself with a sense of being in control, 'captain of my ship' and anticipating his trim self-image. We call that our 'instant yuk' technique. It only takes a couple of seconds and it can be repeated for years."

SALT: A COMMON TRIGGER

It's doubtful you'll ever see someone crazily grab a salt shaker off the table, twist off the cap and start pouring salt down their throat because the urge for the flavor is so strong. The truth is, a sprinkling of salt is all it takes to trigger a binge in some people.

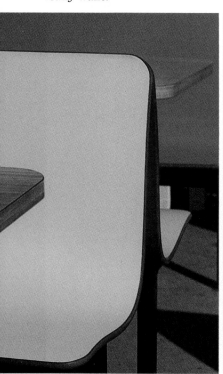
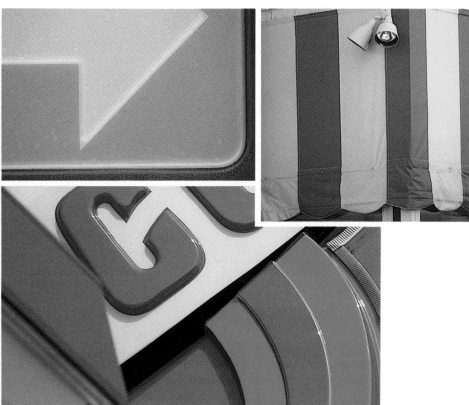

Eda LeShan, a family counselor, wrote about her battle with salt in the book, *Winning the Losing Battle: Why I Will Never Be Fat Again:* "During all the years in which I was in psychotherapy, I assumed that when I went through periods of compulsive eating—when I craved sweets insanely—it was because of some emotional hang-up. . . . but after I'd been [on a salt-free diet] for several weeks, I realized that . . . no matter what my emotional state, I had absolutely no craving for sweets." She cites numerous instances of times salt caused her to binge. "There was to be a dinner right before my speech and I had asked to have fish and vegetables without any salt. I knew as soon as I tasted the food that the chef had not complied; the food was salty, but I ate it because I was hungry . . . That night, when I got back to my hotel room, I became a wild woman, insane for some candy. There was a chocolate mint on each pillow and I ate them immediately; then I started down to the lobby, looking for a candy machine. While I was still in the elevator, I suddenly realized that my craving for sweets was related to salt. The minute I figured it out, I was able to control myself. . . . To lose weight and keep it off, we need to experiment until we figure out which diet is right for us."

Obviously, salt is not the culprit for everyone. But if you are a binge eater, and you suspect that something in your diet is the culprit, try eliminating it the way Eda LeShan gave up salt, and see what happens.

HORMONES CAN CAUSE A BINGE

Some psychologists believe that binging can be caused by an imbalance of hormones brought on by an anxious state of mind. The hormone level is balanced by getting back into a more normal, calm state. Some people achieve this calming effect by eating.

"It's a physiological *and* a psychological problem," says David Margules, Ph.D., a professor in the Temple University psychology department in Philadelphia and president of the National Obesity Research Foundation. Dr. Margules says that stress and tension are directly tied to hormonal shifts. Whether the imbalance is caused by the tension or the tension is caused by the imbalance is not known, according to Dr. Margules. But he does know that normal hormone levels return when a person is calm. Dr. Margules sees a problem in finding relief through food. "The imbalance will usually return after the food has passed through the body," he says.

Because the nature of the problem is so complex, Dr. Margules feels the best way to tackle it is through professional help.

As you can see, there are almost as many genuine causes of binging as there are convenient excuses for stuffing yourself. However, if you can identify your problem and follow through in the steps to correct it, you're well on your way to being binge free forever.

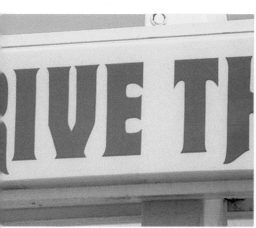
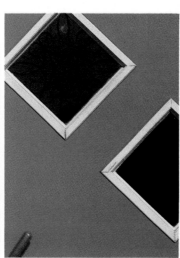
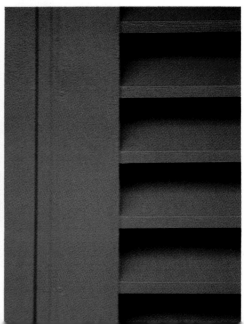

6

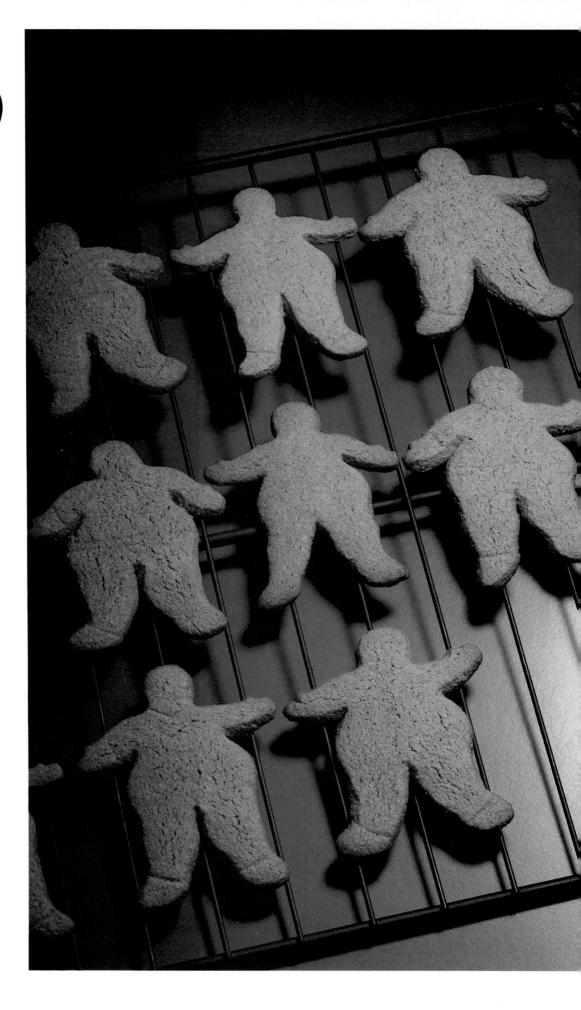

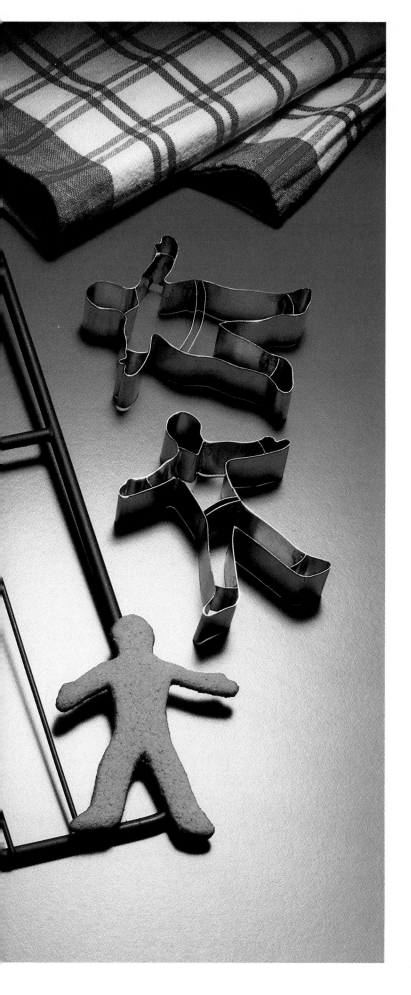

Expert Ideas for Slimmer Eating

It's not what you eat but how you eat that matters most, claim weight-control specialists.

"Imagine if you had a videotape of your life at home from the time you were a child. You could see how your parents fed you, how your grandparents fed you, how food was used in your household. Was it used as a reward? Was it used as punishment? Was it used to console you when you were feeling upset?

"Imagine, if you can, that day when you first toddled over to the refrigerator on your own and opened that door—what did you do with that power? Those are the issues we would like to know more about. Unfortunately, of course, we don't have that videotape."

Those are the words of Dr. Gerard Musante, a behavioral psychologist who directs a weight-loss clinic in Durham, North Carolina. He and other experts believe that successful weight loss is intimately connected to understanding your relationship with food. They believe that the problem isn't only *what* you eat, but when, how, where and why you eat. In short, your behavior around food.

"Being overweight does not occur in a vacuum," says Dr. Musante. "I've never yet had anybody come to me and say, 'I went to bed last night, I was fine, and when I woke up I was fat.' Overweight is really a consequence, a result of a behavior that we've been engaging in over a significant period of time, and that behavior is overeating." These weight-loss experts believe that the solution to the problem is to teach people to change their bad eating habits into good ones. They call this technique behavior modification. And the success rate has been promising.

"Ninety percent of weight-loss programs fail because they *don't* tackle behavior," says Henry Jordan, M.D., director of the Institute for Behavioral Education in King of Prussia, Pennsylvania. But what happens when they do? That's exactly what Rita Yopp Cohen, Ph.D., of the department of psychiatry at the University of Pennsylvania, wanted to find out. She reviewed the results of several weight-loss studies and, not surprisingly, those that involved behavioral techniques came out on top. One particular study compared the weight loss of 102 women who had undergone one of three treatments: behavior therapy, drug therapy or a combination of drug and behavior therapy. At the end of six months the women taking diet pills lost an average of 32 pounds and the combined-treatment group lost an average of 34 pounds. By contrast, the behavior therapy women lost only 24 pounds.

But researchers found a striking reversal of the treatment results at a one-year followup. Behavior-therapy patients "regained far less weight"—4 pounds—while the women who had taken the diet pills regained 18 pounds and the combined-treatment group regained 23½ pounds, almost three-fourths of the weight they lost. At the end of one year, the net weight loss of the behavior-therapy group was the greatest.

This study is typical of many which show that weight loss through behavior modification is slower than with other methods. But, like the tortoise and the hare, slow and steady wins the race.

Ronette Kolotkin, Ph.D., director of the behavioral/psychological component of the Dietary Rehabilitation Center at Duke University Medical Center, has been working with obese patients for years. "It's not always the pattern, but among my most successful patients are some who didn't lose weight for the first two or three months on the program," she says. "Some actually gained weight. But eventually they lost 50 to 60 pounds over the course of two years. It's a lifetime change we're talking about—not a fast solution."

"If you have dieted in the past," says Dr. Musante, "you must ask yourself, why didn't it work? Primarily, it's because what you wanted was a magic formula—and there is no such thing. With those short-sighted methods you become obsessed with how much you weigh: The scale becomes a deity to which you pay homage."

"The truth is, some overweight people are looking for structure," says Kelly Brownell, Ph.D., a behavior specialist at the University

The Overweight Cycle

Being overweight seems to feed upon itself, preying on people's fears and self-doubts. "Behavior is a function of its consequences," says behavioral scientist Gerard Musante, Ph.D. The behavior is excess eating, plus inactivity. The consequences: overweight and withdrawal from social interaction. (The more you gain, the less you get around.) That leads to negative feelings and self-deprecation—which make you eat more. "It's an insidious cycle," says Dr. Musante, "and the way to break it is to alter the behavior."

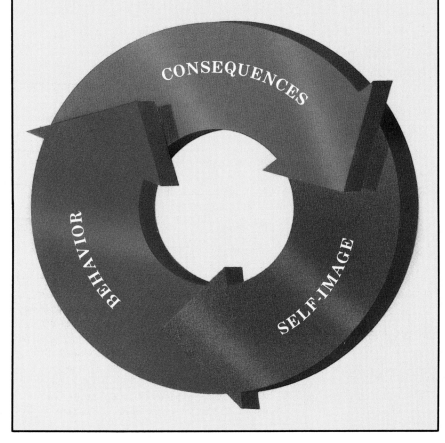

of Pennsylvania. "A rigid diet offers structure, yes, but with impermanent results. Behavior modification offers a structure to behavior—with lasting results. Eventually, the person who loses weight through changing his behavior and restructuring his lifestyle will gain a sense of control."

To help you get started on your plan of control—to reform your own attitude about food once and for all—we talked to the nation's top behavior modification experts about their most successful techniques. Here's what they recommend.

KEEP A FOOD DIARY

Imagine a salesperson without an appointment book. Or executives who don't write down the meetings they have to attend. In fact, think of any busy person trying to successfully meet the responsibilities and challenges of the day without some kind of written record. It would be next to impossible!

Well, weight loss is a challenge, too. You have to know what you're eating and what you plan to eat. And the best way to do that is to keep an accurate record—a food diary.

At the University of Pennsylvania obesity clinic, Dr. Brownell and his colleagues, Albert Stunkard, M.D., and Dr. Thomas Wadden, put a great deal of emphasis on the diet diary. "The food diary serves a number of very valuable functions," explains Dr. Brownell. "I know people who have kept a food diary for ten years. It can get to be a nuisance, but almost all of our patients, after they've lost weight, tell us later that the food diary was the most useful tool of behavior modification. I'm not saying that you have to keep a diary for ten years—although those people who did tended to maintain a good weight loss. There are many, many people who keep a food diary for a while and eventually quit keeping it once they've begun to do well on the program."

What does keeping a food diary entail? Basically, it means writing down everything you eat every day

and at what time you eat it. Most of the top behavior-modification clinics in the country encourage people to elaborate even more. "We have people write down everything they put into their mouths—along with when they ate it, with whom, what mood they were in, how hungry they felt, the degree of appetite and so on," says Maria Simonson, Ph.D., director of the Health, Weight and Stress Clinic at Johns Hopkins University Hospital in Baltimore. "At the end of two weeks—even without being on a diet— they've usually lost 1 to 3 pounds."

THE 'REAL' YOU SHOWS THROUGH

No diet, no diet pills—just a record of you and food. How can such a

DIET DIARY

NAME:
DATE:

FOOD	TIME	PLACE	FEELINGS	ACTIVITY	CALORIES
BREAKFAST	10 AM	KITCHEN TABLE	RELAXED	CONVERSATION	
2 FRIED EGGS					198
2 SLICES W/W TOAST					112
2 TSP BUTTER					68
2 SLICES BACON					88
COFFEE W/ SKIM MILK	10:30	KITCH. TABLE	BORED	READING THE PAPER	11
LUNCH	2 PM	KITCHEN TABLE	CAREFREE & PEPPY	NOTHING	
1 CUP PORK AND BEAN SOUP					168
3 OUNCES MUSHROOMS					57
SALAD W/ TABLESPOON OF DRESSING					25 / 78
DINNER	4 PM	MOTHER'S DINING ROOM	ON EDGE	CONVERSATION	
1 CUP CHICKEN RICE SOUP					
2 OUNCES ROAST CHICKEN					48 104
1 OZ. MEATBALL					57
1 OZ. SAUSAGE					134
½ CUP RICOTTA CHEESE					100
½ CUP MACARONI					78
¼ CUP SPAGHETTI SAUCE					55
TEA WITH LEMON	6 PM	MOTHER'S DINING ROOM	FEEL BETTER	CONV.	5
COFFEE W/ SKIM MILK	8 PM	AUNT'S HOUSE	CHEERY	TALKING	11
COFFEE W/ SKIM MILK	8:30 PM	"	"	"	11

EXERCISE	TIME	PLACE	FEELING	NUMBER OF MINUTES
WALKING	1 PM	NEAR HOME	FEEL GOOD	30 MIN.

This is an example of a page from a diet diary like those kept by patients at the University of Pennsylvania obesity clinic. Doctors there and at other clinics feel that keeping a diary is one of the most useful tools—if not *the* most useful— in coming to grips with your eating problems. Your diet diary can be as simple or complicated as you'd like it to be, but doctors recommend that you at least record the time and place of the meal. Recording your activity and what you are feeling at the moment, however, can make you aware of why you eat the way you do. The doctors also feel a diet diary is useful even after you lose weight because it helps you stay in control.

simple device work? It works in several ways, the experts tell us. First of all, it makes you aware of how much you're actually eating. According to Isobel Contento, Ph.D., an associate professor of nutrition and education at Teachers College, Columbia University. Studies show that "people who eat a lot tend to underestimate the amount of food they eat, while people who eat a little tend to overestimate the amount of food they eat," she says. "When it comes to food intake it is difficult to be accurate."

Aside from sheer quantity, a diary points up the quality of foods you eat. If breakfast is often a cup of coffee and a doughnut, lunch a hamburger and a soft drink and dinner a small salad followed by a bowl of ice cream, plus a late-night snack of pretzels or potato chips, the weight reducer can be reminded in black and white that this kind of diet is definitely lacking in good nutrition.

Even so, our experts say you should never divide food into categories of "good" and "bad." Dr. Brownell explains, "In our program, there are no forbidden fruits, no foods that the dieter must *never* eat. Saying 'I'll never eat cake again' sets the dieter up for failure when they 'succumb' to having a piece at someone's birthday party. Eating something that's a no-no in the dieter's book will lead to self-blame and a sense of having failed again in a weight-loss attempt."

At the University of Pennsylvania clinic, the focus is on limiting calories at a healthy level—one where the dieters can still enjoy their favorite foods, but with an eye to optimum nutrition. "We ascribe to nutritional principles above all," Dr. Brownell says. His colleague Dr. Wadden puts it this way: "The idea is not to deprive yourself of the foods you crave, but to be able to control yourself when faced with those foods."

A food diary also can reveal essential personal truths about your eating patterns—not just preferences for certain foods but times of the day or days of the week (such as the weekend) when you tend to overeat or eat out of sheer habit.

"By seeing your eating patterns," says Dr. Simonson, "you can eliminate some unnecessary eating. For example, the diary may show a person that he's eating a snack every afternoon even when he doesn't really feel hungry."

A diary can also help detect some psychological reasons behind your overeating. You may notice, for example, that you overeat every single time you have lunch with your mother. You love her dearly, but somehow seeing her transports you back to the days of "Clean your plate or you can't have dessert."

Discovering your personal eating patterns through the pages of a diet diary is a major step you can take toward your goal of permanent weight loss. It will help you understand why you overeat. Your diary can serve as your "personal warning system" to tip you off *before* your eating gets out of control. Once you have taken this step, the next one, becoming the master of your own eating habits, will come more easily.

DISCOVER YOUR FOOD CUES

The path to weight loss is fraught with land mines and booby traps. A menu with beautiful pictures of food is one type of trap: It makes a direct appeal to your stomach, which then overrides any will power you might have. Fortunately, most of us don't have to go into restaurants every day. But there is one trap we do have to encounter daily—in fact, many times daily. It's the home refrigerator.

How often do you go into the kitchen and fling open the doors of the cabinet underneath the sink—the one where all the cleansers are—just for the heck of it? Most likely, you hardly ever do. Now how many times do you walk into the kitchen, fling open the refrigerator door and mindlessly snatch something from the shelf? Well, you don't have to answer that one. You probably get the point. The refrigerator is one of those food cues, something that signals a behavior in you that makes you want to eat,

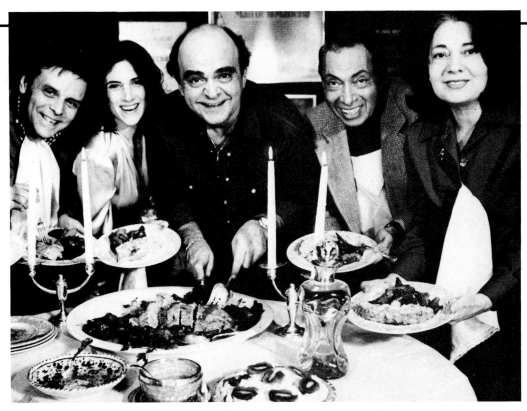

whether you planned to or not. To gain control over your eating behavior, you need to cultivate new habits and strategies to cope with "the enemy." It may well mean you need to go on a search-and-destroy mission around your house. That doesn't mean you should blow up the refrigerator or the TV, if you love to eat while watching it. The changes you must make in your behavior and your surroundings are subtle ones—ones you can adjust to and live with for the rest of your life.

For example, let's see what you can do to deal with the refrigerator. Obviously, one answer would be to have two refrigerators—one that you could put out of the way, perhaps in the cellar, that would contain items of temptation like ice cream or soft drinks. (This, of course, is assuming that you keep these items because someone else in the family wants them. If they're for you, you should throw them away.) Unfortunately, most people don't have this option. So here's where a little strategy comes in.

Load the front of the refrigerator with fruits, vegetables and meat-and-potato-type leftovers. The half-eaten lemon chiffon pie should be pushed way in the back and hidden from view. The storage

shelves on the inside of your refrigerator door should be restricted to holding items like eggs and butter. As for the freezer compartment, put ice cream or similar snacks in the back—behind the frozen meats and vegetables and completely out of sight. The old adage, "Out of sight, out of mind" can work quite well with your appetite.

Stage and television actor James Coco, who lost 110 pounds while attending Dr. Musante's Structure House, credits his success to being able to pin down several of his danger traps. "I found that whenever I talked on the telephone, I munched on nuts," he recalls. "There was always a bowl of them next to the phone. At parties, I always found myself next to the buffet table. And I ate incredible amounts of food while I was cooking—I love to cook. It took wearing a surgical mask to break me of that habit!"

THE PATH TO SELF-CONTROL

Behavioral therapists refer to control over eating cues as "stimulus control and environmental management." Here are some of their most

That's a new body you see on stage and film star James Coco. He's finally kicked the losing-eating-gaining habit that had him struggling with obesity all his adult life. He's a thinner man today after having shed 110 pounds while attending the behavior modification clinic, Structure House, in Durham, North Carolina. In fact, he's so impressed with his achievement, he's written a book, *The James Coco Diet,* based on what he learned at the clinic. Here he samples some of his favorite diet recipes with Structure House grads, including his coauthor, Marion Paone, far right. It goes to show—anybody can lose weight!

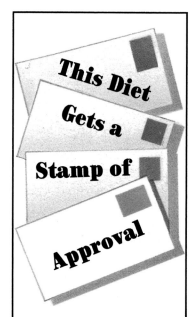

This Diet Gets a Stamp of Approval

Stanford University researchers have found a unique—and successful—way to get faculty members and their families to lose weight: They put them in a mail-order weight-loss program.

"People respond to 15 weekly packets and mail in weekly reports," says Joel Killen, Ph.D., "They write about their urges, identify problems, describe tough situations and how they plan to handle them. We strive to help people develop problem-solving skills, to avoid getting overcome by eating urges."

The program has been a big success.

useful recommendations:

• Make eating a "pure" experience. Eat only at the kitchen table or dining room table, and always use a place setting. Never eat in any room other than the kitchen or dining room. And never eat while standing up. (Remember the refrigerator habit?) Also, says Dr. Stunkard, "avoid pairing your eating with other activities." Many an extra calorie is put on by eating while reading, watching TV, walking, driving, cooking and so on.

• Shop wisely. The "out of sight, out of mind" adage works well here, too. If you don't buy it, you won't be tempted to eat it.

• Store food wisely. Keep food only in the kitchen and pantry. Place high-calorie items in hard-to-reach places, on the highest shelves or behind other foods in the refrigerator. Put the cake saver away with the pots and pans until you need it. (Seeing it empty may spur you to fill it.) And don't use glass jars to store brownies— fill the jars with herb teas and dried beans instead.

• Make use of signs—whatever works for you—on the refrigerator, your desk or wherever necessary.

• Be on guard at social gatherings. "When people are in social situations— when they're happy and celebrating and feeling particularly gregarious—they may overeat, especially if they've been having alcohol," says Dr. Wadden. "Alcohol decreases our inhibitions, which include our inhibitions toward eating." Dr. Wadden suggests eating something *before* you go to the party, such as a salad or light sandwich. He also recommends making the first drink a glass of water. That way you won't be so hungry or thirsty soon after you arrive. He also cautions selectiveness in choosing party snacks. Many tend to be salty, which can encourage even more drinking and eating. "There's no question that

increased salt intake can cause you to want to drink more and consume more," he says.

DEVELOP NEW EATING SKILLS

Did you ever try to change your posture for the better—to square your shoulders, lift your chest and stand tall? Your resolution probably lasted about a day, if that. And then your body slumped back into its habitual mold. Maybe not the best way to sit and stand, but *your* way.

Old habits die hard. They seem chiseled into our personalities by years of repetition, as much a part of us as our skin. And bad eating habits are no exception. You try to change them but before you know it they've snagged you again—you're in their power. The only way to conquer them is to square off, look 'em in the eye, see them for what they really are and pull a few fast ones before they get you first.

When breaking bad eating habits, it's best to meet them on their own turf—at the table. Here are some new skills to practice so that eating doesn't get out of hand. They're very simple, yet extraordinarily effective.

Slow Down! It was another one of those "sneaky" experiments. Fifty-five women who had lost weight through behavior modification and 26 women who had never gone through such a program were told they would be entering a "tasting room" to rate the flavor of three different crackers. But behind a one-way screen was a group of researchers who were there to observe the real purpose of the experiment: to see how much each woman would eat in a 7-minute period. As the researchers anticipated, the women who had learned their eating habits through behavior modification ate less than the women who hadn't. This observation leads to an interesting insight into the weight-loss story. It suggests that *eating less is associated with eating slowly.*

Experts feel that, in general, overweight people eat faster than people of normal weight. And there

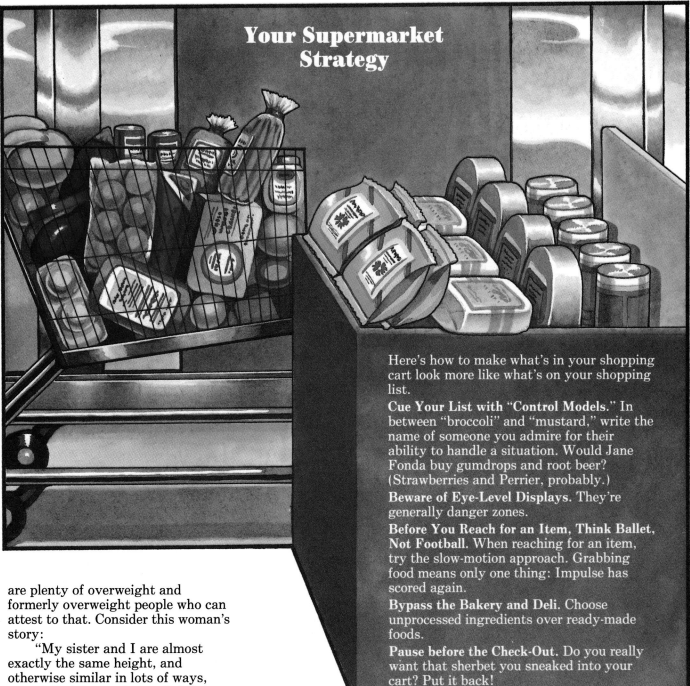

Your Supermarket Strategy

Here's how to make what's in your shopping cart look more like what's on your shopping list.

Cue Your List with "Control Models." In between "broccoli" and "mustard," write the name of someone you admire for their ability to handle a situation. Would Jane Fonda buy gumdrops and root beer? (Strawberries and Perrier, probably.)

Beware of Eye-Level Displays. They're generally danger zones.

Before You Reach for an Item, Think Ballet, Not Football. When reaching for an item, try the slow-motion approach. Grabbing food means only one thing: Impulse has scored again.

Bypass the Bakery and Deli. Choose unprocessed ingredients over ready-made foods.

Pause before the Check-Out. Do you really want that sherbet you sneaked into your cart? Put it back!

are plenty of overweight and formerly overweight people who can attest to that. Consider this woman's story:

"My sister and I are almost exactly the same height, and otherwise similar in lots of ways, except that I was always fighting an extra 25 or 30 pounds on and off. Vivian never had a weight problem—and probably never will. First of all, she'd have to spend 24 hours a day eating to do that, not because her metabolism is so fast, but because she eats so slowly. Even when we were kids, she was always the last to finish eating. If someone tries to hurry her along, saying something like, 'Let's just grab a bite before we go,' she'll put on her coat and say, 'Let's go now.' She'd rather not eat at all than eat in a rush.

"After I had my baby, I was left with a lot of 'baby fat' of my own—and it didn't drop off, either. So I enrolled in a behavior modification and exercise program at my company, and lost 50 pounds over a year. It's amazing—I'm down to my high school weight now and really don't think about food or gaining weight any more. But when I sit down to eat, I do think about Vivian, even though she's 2,000 miles away, and I *make that meal last.*"

Eating slowly is a technique with a particularly nice side effect: It allows you to savor food. In his book, *I Almost Feel Thin,* Dr. Stunkard quotes one of his patients, a young college woman who had struggled with overeating for years: "A couple of nights ago, when I was studying, I went into my roommate's room and took a cookie, just *one cookie,* from a box that she had there. I ate it very slowly, chewing it carefully and tasting every part of it. And then I went back in my room to study. I was in absolute awe of myself—was this the same Mary O'Brien who two months ago wouldn't have been able to stop at *ten cookies,* let alone one; who would have eaten the whole box and then another one if it was there?"

But how do you learn to eat slowly when you have spent your life chowing down like you were in a pie-eating contest? Our experts recommend these three tips.

1. Chew food *thoroughly* before swallowing.
2. Count each mouthful of food and lay your fork or spoon down after every bite.

The Psychology of Place Settings

Did you ever wolf down a hamburger you tore from a paper wrapper? Or do you find yourself piling your new lime green china with seconds and even thirds? If so, it may not be the food alone that's whetting your appetite. It could have a lot to do with what you're putting your food *on.* Weight-loss experts believe that appetite reacts strongly to place settings and some ways of setting the table can actually help us eat less. One method that researchers have found to work well is the Japanese setting—small portions on small plates— such as the one pictured at left below. "Their dishes can look like a bouquet on a plate, they are so beautifully arranged," says Maria Simonson, Ph.D. "And in actuality, the food in front of you is about one-third of the amount that you might otherwise think you'd be satisfied with."

The formal place setting, such as the one in the second photo, also helps appease the appetite. "In general, people eat less in a formal setting than a rustic or family-style setting," she says. You feel less free to help yourself to more, you eat

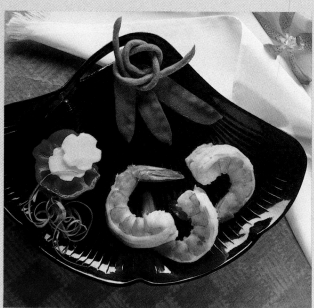
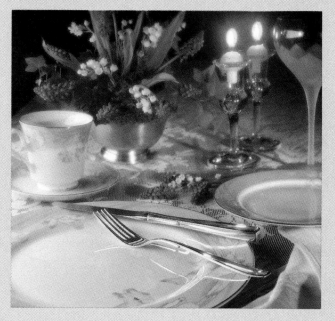

3. Be the last to start eating and the last to finish. "When you are eating with other people, talk, rearrange your napkin, cut your meat into tiny pieces . . . stall any way you can to be the last person to start eating," says Dr. Brownell. "During the meal maintain a pace that will guarantee that you are the last one finished."

Think about it. If eating is to be a pleasurable activity, it deserves your time and concentration.

Stick to Your Own Plate. Many overweight people are compulsive plate cleaners—and they don't stop at their own plate, either. In a house where there are young children (who are notorious for their erratic eating patterns), parents sometimes get into the habit of "picking" at their children's leftovers. For a person prone to weight gain, this can be a dangerous practice. A roll of plastic wrap kept in a very handy place (perhaps even on the table) will help solve that problem: Simply wrap the plate and put it in the refrigerator—immediately. Or give it to the dog. Whatever you do, don't leave it on the table.

more slowly and pay more attention to the manner in which you eat in a formal setting.

As for pasta, Dr. Simonson says it's best to serve it in a bowl with a raised edge, as in the third photo, instead of on a plate. "It will give you a sense of satisfaction, even though the same amount of spaghetti on a plate won't look like enough."

As for plates in general, the best types to use are those that are plain in the center with raised colored borders, such as those in the last photo. They, too, give the impression of having more on the plate. As for colors, pastels, beige and plain white are among the best.

So, what should you avoid? Splashy colors such as bright blues, violets, bright yellow and lime green, says Dr. Simonson. They stimulate the appetite. So, too, do pewter and wooden plates. "In our experiments, we found that people ate more off those than silver or vermeil plates," she says. "Perhaps you feel because it's primitive, you can pig out more."

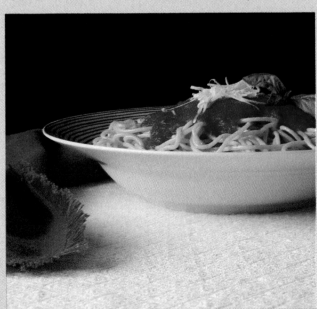

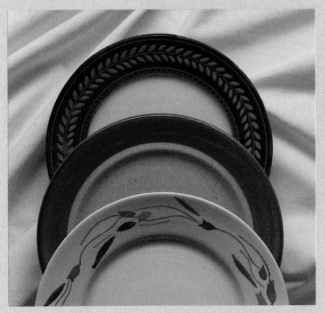

Aside from laziness (that is, avoiding stashing leftovers because it requires effort), the reasons behind plate cleaning often stem from guilt feelings that go back to childhood. James Coco recalls, "Before I began to deal with behavior modification and changing my lifestyle, there never was a leftover in my house. I really was the sort of person who would go gung-ho and clean out the cupboards and the refrigerator and then wake up at 2 in the morning, find nine peppercorns and eat them. And I realized it had something to do with growing up Italian, and also being told at the table, 'Finish your food—people are starving all over the world,' and I'd think, 'Oh, my God, I can't let people starve, I'd better eat my food.' And one day I realized that people were still starving—but I was getting fat."

Leave a Bit Behind. It may sound like heresy, but to break yourself of compulsive plate cleaning, practice leaving food on your plate. Some successful weight reducers say they now leave just a mouthful—as a matter of course. Also, learn to police your own portion control by dishing out your meal from the stove directly to the plate. If some family members want seconds, all they have to do is go back to the kitchen. Serving food "family style," with all that extra food heaped into serving bowls on the table, only encourages latent plate cleaning, experts say.

PLAN AND PREPLAN

There's something very satisfying about the ritual of eating a nice meal at the table. Eating ravioli right out of the baking pan while standing next to the kitchen sink, for instance, may provide a pleasant taste experience, but somehow, something is missing.

"Take a look at a Japanese meal, for example," says Dr. Simonson. "It's served artfully—it looks sculptured almost—which makes it more appetizing and also more filling. They take the time to

structure their meals, making food so desirable to the eye and tongue that the satiety value is quite high—though actually, the food in front of you is about one-third of the amount you might otherwise think you'd be satisfied with. And they don't eat much between meals."

It's not surprising that some behavioral therapists blame haphazard, unplanned eating as a primary cause of overweight. Dr. Musante believes so strongly in structured eating that he calls his North Carolina clinic Structure House. Structured eating is breakfast, lunch and dinner—the meals we take to fulfill our basic nutritional needs. Anything beyond that he considers *un*structured.

After 12 years of research, working with hundreds of patients, Dr. Musante and his staff came to the conclusion that every episode of unstructured eating is the result of one of three things: habit, boredom or stress.

Eating out of habit rather than hunger is quite common, says Dr. Musante, because it is an automatic response—something we learned in childhood. "Anyone can be subjected to this, including people who have never had a weight problem, because we're all creatures of habit," he says.

Boredom, however, is a little more insidious. "As soon as people gain weight, they stop doing things," he says. "They've decreased the repertoire of behaviors they can engage in; they're limited in the ways they can entertain themselves." But they know that one way they can still entertain themselves is with food. Because they have nothing to do, or because they don't want to do the things they liked to do when they were thin, they eat.

In the stress situation, Dr. Musante says, people use food as a tranquilizer. "You're upset, you eat, you feel better. What it all comes down to is changing a lifestyle that is characterized by habit, boredom and stress."

At Structure House, one way they get people to make these changes is by getting them in the habit of planning all their meals well in advance. "We're not saying you can't engage in unstructured eating,

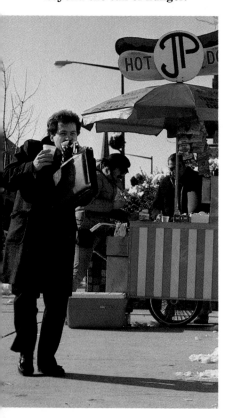

Eating on the run can easily lead to "eating amnesia," says Henry Jordan, M.D., of the Institute for Behavioral Education, outside Philadelphia. "People who eat too fast or eat while doing something else are attempting to be efficient. But if you ask them an hour later what they ate, they often can't remember. Also, fast eaters are overeaters," says Dr. Jordan. That's because the body cues that signal satiety travel slowly from stomach to brain, so fast eaters don't receive the critical message "Stop! I'm full!" until they've eaten well above and beyond the call of hunger.

but that if you do, be aware of it," says Dr. Musante.

How far in advance are we talking about? Many people find that planning their meals about a week in advance works the best. It also helps to buy only as much food as you'll need for each meal.

ERASE BLACK-AND-WHITE THINKING

By now you know how important it is to be careful of what you're eating when you're trying to lose weight. But there's another dictum for dieters that's equally important: Be careful of what you're *thinking.*

"One of the most damaging patterns of thinking is on-and-off thinking—what I call black-and-white thinking," says Dr. Wadden. "The biggest problem dieters have is they have such high expectations of themselves that they can't possibly meet these expectations." The result: They abandon the diet.

"They're not so much perfectionists, but rather people who buy into the body image promoted by the media—they buy into the thought that they should be thin," he explains. "A lot of people think that if they don't achieve their goal, anything short of the goal is a failure. It's a very dichotomized thinking pattern: You've either succeeded or you've failed. We try to help people quantify success and say if you lost 2 pounds that it's terrific. It wasn't the 2½ pounds you had your heart set on, but it's still a great success."

Overeating in itself does not lead to negative feelings, explains Dr. Brownell. It's how a person *perceives* the overeating that matters the most. For example, there are some overweight people who would respond to eating an extra-large piece of cheesecake with this range of thinking: "Oh, what a pig I am; I'm so disgusted with myself I don't deserve to lose weight." Dr. Brownell calls this a "catastrophic statement"—a value judgment that leads to negative feelings.

"However, there are all kinds of ways to look positively upon events—even overeating," he says.

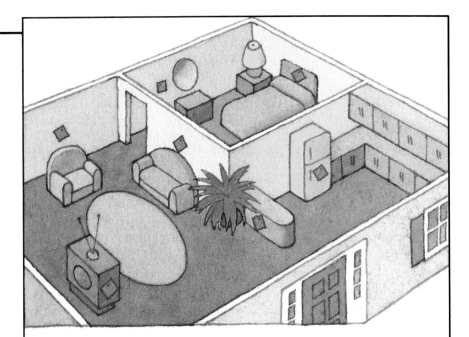

The Road to Success Is Well Marked

There's nothing like a caution sign on a dull stretch of highway to rouse you just as you are slipping into a semihypnotic state. Likewise, "road signs" placed in your home can jolt you out of a potentially destructive situation by reminding you of your weight-loss goals. The refrigerator is an obvious signboard, but don't stop there. On a kitchen cabinet, you might want to cue yourself to "Eat at the table, please." If you need to walk more, signs like "Want to lose some weight, right now?" and "Home of the world's champion walker" can go on the coat closet door. In the bathroom might go the reminder "Each day I am a thinner person"; near the TV, "Have a tall, cool glass of water"; in the family room, "Knit three rows of that sweater, now!" And don't forget "Think thin." Go for upbeat messages—nothing self-deprecating. Signs like "Hold it, Fatso" only damage the psyche at a time when it most needs uplifting.

A statement such as, "Well, that was an extra 300 calories. I'll have to take a nice, long walk after dinner tonight to make up for it," works much, much better.

So, how can you stop being so down on yourself? One way is to state your feelings out loud. It helps show how silly they really can be. Dr. Wadden says this works well in his weight-loss clinics. "In a group

(continued on page 100)

Self-Hypnosis

Hypnosis for weight loss? It's not hocus-pocus. Physicians and weight-control therapists are finding hypnosis remarkably helpful as a way to reinforce new, healthy eating habits.

If this sounds suspicious to you, it's probably because you associate hypnosis with dangling pocketwatches and suspicious-looking men with bushy eyebrows. But hypnosis is something you can use yourself, quite safely and effectively. Basically, self-hypnosis is a form of deep relaxation that allows you to enter a state of altered consciousness. You do enter a trance, yes, but it's not a sleepy state—your mind is actually at peak awareness, even though your eyes are closed. It's something akin to being so absorbed in a book that it takes several seconds before you realize the phone's been ringing. Of course, just as you eventually put down your book and become alert to your real surroundings, you also will come out of a hypnotic state with ease, feeling refreshed as well.

There are 3 basic phases of a self-hypnosis session. The first is to induce the hypnotic state itself, usually through some type of relaxation technique. Once you are deeply relaxed, your mind will be unusually receptive to the positive suggestions you give it. You are then ready for the "work" phase, when you focus on changing an aspect of your behavior and developing a positive outlook on yourself in relation to eating, exercise and losing weight in general.

During this phase (which is much shorter than the induction phase), you will make suggestions to yourself. But to be useful, those suggestions must involve vivid imagery and focus on just one idea. Saying to yourself, "I'm going to start walking for a half hour every day and eat fewer snacks" simply won't work well. It's far better to choose a *situation* before you begin hypnosis and then imagine yourself in that situation, responding in a positive, rational fashion. For

example, if you have trouble getting motivated to exercise, your "work" phase may sound like this:

"It's 5:15 and I've just walked in the front door. My dog is wagging his tail, eager for our daily walk. I'm changing into my sneakers and sweat suit, feeling good about the fact that the pants are feeling so baggy these days. The dog and I are outside now, walking briskly in the cool, fresh air. Golden leaves crackle underfoot, and I hear Canada geese honking long before I can see their perfect 'V' formation. I'm burning calories with each step I take, and feeling wonderfully refreshed. It's great to be outside after sitting at a desk all day."

After "playing" that scenario about twice a week for a few weeks, you will likely find it easier to go home and immediately don sweats instead of plunking down into an easy chair. But suppose that after your walk, you discover yourself drinking a quart of root beer. Your next hypnotic "work" phase might go like this: "I've just come home from my daily walk and I feel fantastically invigorated from the fresh air and the exercise. I'm thirsty, too, and my body needs water to replenish fluids. A cool, clear glass of spring water will taste delicious. It is exactly what I desire now. I am filling a glass and drinking it, slowly, and it quenches my thirst and refreshes me completely." You get the idea. Each scenario should be tailored to suit your needs and liberally infused with self-statements of feeling good about the weight-loss progress you have made, no matter how much.

The last phase, the conclusion, involves breaking the trance slowly. Counting backward from 10 to 0 works well.

There are so many negative influences on our eating habits—from TV's barrage to people who say, "What's a few extra pounds?" —that we need to provide positive influences as a counterbalance. Hypnosis can do just that.

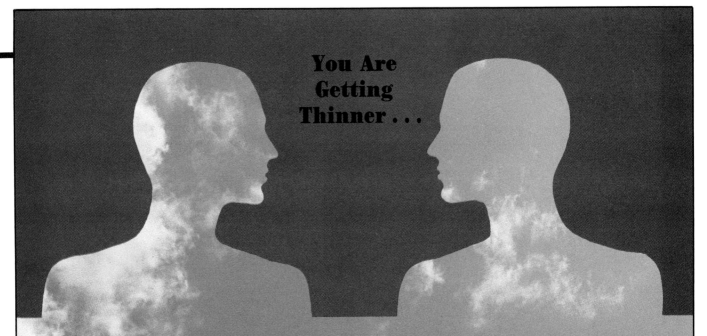

You Are Getting Thinner . . .

There are many, many ways to induce hypnosis, but this technique is fairly easy, straightforward and effective. Since dinnertime is a prime time to overeat, the scenario described during the "work" phase focuses on that problem.

Induction. Lie down in a quiet, comfortable place, like on your bed. Take a couple of deep breaths to start. When you exhale, feel yourself relax. Let your stomach expand with each inhalation and exhale slowly. You are breathing normally now, and with each exhalation you can feel your legs growing limp and pleasantly warm. You can feel all your bones actually settling deeper into your bed as your thighs and buttocks and back muscles relax.

Now the day's tensions are being drained from your chest, your arms, your shoulders. And as you feel your scalp and your face relax, your eyes close quite naturally. Your head feels quite heavy. You're beautifully relaxed now and it feels wonderful.

Now you are going to count backward from 10 to 0, and when you reach 0, you will be much, much more relaxed than you are now. 10 . . . 9 . . . deeper and deeper . . . 8 . . . 7 . . . 6 . . . 5 . . . 4 . . . 3 . . . 2 . . . 1 . . . 0. You are now in a very, very deep state of relaxation. And you are going to become even more relaxed, much more relaxed than ever before.

Imagine a time when you were incredibly happy and tranquil. Perhaps it was a quiet afternoon at the beach. You are there now. The sun warms your body as a cool breeze caresses your cheeks. You say to yourself, "I feel deliciously warm . . . I've never felt so peaceful." You give yourself up completely to the beauty of this moment . . . and as you do so, you realize that you are now in a deep trance.

"Work" Phase. Next, visualize yourself sitting at the dinner table. Your plate is filled, but not heaped, with some of your favorite foods. You are eating slowly, savoring the aroma, the texture and the flavor of each bite as you chew and swallow. Slowly, as you eat, your sense of satisfaction grows until you are finished. Your stomach still doesn't feel quite full, which is perfectly normal because it takes about 20 minutes after you have stopped eating before your food gives you a sensation of fullness. You tell yourself, "I have eaten all that my body needs for perfect energy and well-being, and all that I really want to eat. My mouth will feel relaxed and serene throughout the evening." You leave the table and go into another room to pursue a favorite activity. You can see yourself doing that activity, while at the same time, the feeling of fullness increases until, after 20 minutes, you feel quite satisfied. There is enough food to take you easily through to the next morning.

Conclusion. Take several deep breaths. As you inhale, you become more and more alert to your immediate surroundings. You realize where you are, and begin slowly counting backward from 10. Take a breath with each number and be aware that as you do so, you are becoming increasingly alert. At 7, your eyelids are becoming lighter. As you reach 5 and then 4, you become increasingly aware of your hands and your legs touching the surface they're on and it will be good to be fully awake again. Your eyelids now have an irresistible urge to open and just as you reach 1, they do open and you are fully alert.

session, for instance, one person says to herself and the others, 'I really screwed up badly last night. I ate 100 calories of potato chips above what I said I was going to eat. I feel like a failure.' Then I might say to a member of the group, 'Would you please tell her she's a failure because she ate too many potato chips?' When the group harangues her, it sounds ridiculous, and we end up laughing. We try to give people some objective perspective. Then we give them a

statement they can say to themselves that's more reasonable and more helpful."

Putting all this into practice isn't easy at first. You've got to give it time. "In behavior modification," says Dr. Brownell, "you must realize first that the changes won't come overnight. It takes a lot of practice to get over those negative thoughts and feelings that have occurred many times."

Remember, every time you make a nasty statement about yourself and your eating habits, you may be pushing your diet efforts back a step or two. That fact should be enough to make you want to "think positive."

PICK A PARTNER

How often do you hear someone lament that they didn't go to the movie the night before or missed the baseball game because they "didn't have anybody to go with"? Making an event more interesting or fun is a lot easier when it involves more than one person. The same goes for dieting. While it may be stretching it a bit to say dieting is fun, it's sometimes a task that's a lot easier to tackle if there is someone around for support.

Diet experts say the support can come from anyone—a fellow dieter, a friend at work or a spouse. For some people a support group is the answer.

"Of course there is no rule that applies to every person," says Dr. Brownell, who wrote a book on the subject, *The Partnership Diet Program*. "For some people it helps to enlist the aid of a spouse; other people find that they need to get away from home—to a clinical setting—to break the cycle of overweight.

"Eventually, though," he says, "most people find it easier to lose weight and keep it off if the environment they live in supports their efforts. That's why spouses are important. They can make it easier to comply with the program of behavior modification. They help reinforce the technique of the weight-loss program."

Help Yourself to Self-Help

Finding some help or moral support in your weight-loss efforts may be as easy as checking your telephone book. But don't fall for the get-thin-quick centers—look instead to self-help groups that have established solid reputations for helping people lose weight and keep it off.

• Weight Watchers members meet weekly to weigh in and talk about obesity, nutrition, exercise and behavioral skills. They've even developed a brand of low-calorie cuisine, which is available in most supermarkets.

• TOPS (Take Off Pounds Sensibly) is a strictly noncommercial, nonprofit group, whose speakers are often people who've lost substantial amounts of weight through the TOPS program; clubs vie with each other to take off the most weight and win medals.

• Overeaters Anonymous is a support group for people who have a problem with uncontrolled eating.

The national headquarters for each group is given below:

Weight Watchers International, Inc.
800 Community Drive
Manhasset, NY 11030

TOPS Club, Inc.
4575 South 5th Street
P.O. Box 07489
Milwaukee, WI 53207-0489

Overeaters Anonymous
2190 West 190th Street
Torrance, CA 90504

WEIGHT LOSS: A REWARDING EXPERIENCE

There's this story about a doctor who worked out a deal with his music-loving patient. The patient was overweight and desperately wanted to get thin. His doctor convinced the man to turn over to him all his precious records, which would be returned only if he lost at least a pound each week. For every pound, a record was returned. If no weight was lost the doctor chose a record from the collection for himself. Eventually, the patient won his collection back. He got his reward.

Obviously, there's a lot of room to be creative in devising ways to reward your weight loss. It could go the route of a new dress when you hit size 9 or a vacation trip after you drop 50 pounds. Those "finish line" rewards are nice—a real treat for a job well done.

However, there are some behavior therapists who feel such rewards are too long in coming. They feel more immediate rewards have more impact.

"Every obese person has had some experience with rewards, but usually they have been too infrequent and too long delayed" says Dr. Stunkard in his book. "As one housewife put it, 'My husband might offer to buy me a car if I lost 50 pounds. And I might knock myself out and lose 30 pounds, which is a lot of weight. But what did it get me—half a car? I got nothing.'"

For his group sessions, Dr. Stunkard and his colleagues "devised a system which awarded the patient a certain number of points immediately after each of the activities we were trying to encourage: record keeping, counting bites and swallows and so on. These effectively provided immediate reward, and as we gained experience, we added increasingly sophisticated schedules, such as doubling the number of points earned when a patient devised and performed an activity which was an alternative to eating in the face of strong temptation."

You can devise such a reward system for yourself. For every pound you lose, for instance, you could give yourself a point and for every five points earned you could indulge yourself with something that is non-food oriented. Perhaps after five points you'd get a massage, after ten you could see a Broadway show. Of course, you could still save a big reward for the final goal. It'll help you treat your weight-loss program like a game—a game in which you're bound to end up the winner.

How can you be sure you'll be able to move along peak by small peak toward your final goal? By changing your bad habits into good—by following the steps of behavior modification. After a time they'll become second nature. As Dr. Wadden puts it, your new habits will become "as routine as brushing your teeth."

Going for the (Weight Loss) Cure

How do you know when it's time to check into a special clinic for your weight problem? "People usually come to us after all other weight-loss methods have failed," says Kelly Brownell, Ph.D., of the University of Pennsylvania. His colleague Thomas Wadden, Ph.D., points out, "There are a couple of good signs to go by. Repeated starts and failures are a clue. If you chronically diet and chronically gain back weight, it's clear you haven't changed your eating and exercise habits to maintain weight loss. How you are motivated to change your behavior is another question—an individual one."

One of their patients, Rich Binetsky, who lost 75 pounds, says, "I began to ask myself, 'What am I going to do—yo-yo all my life?' Then my wife told me that my son had asked her if people who are overweight live as long as others, or do they die earlier? That was the straw that was needed. I went to talk to Dr. Wadden, and before I knew it, I was in the program."

Clinics that meet weekly for 6 months cost between $250 and $1,000; live-in clinics obviously cost more—about $200 to $400 per week plus registration and housing fees.

Overweight Children

If you weigh too much, there's a 40 percent chance your kids do, too. And if you and your spouse are both overweight, the probability increases to 80 percent. On the other hand, if neither parent is obese, there's only a 10 percent chance that your children will be overweight.

Without a doubt, genetics play a role in body stature. But statistics say that inborn endocrine problems account for a mere 3 percent of all obesity in children, and rare syndromes are responsible for just 2 percent. Most often, a tubby child is a victim of overnutrition coupled with a lack of exercise. In other words, fat kids are eating too much (or are being fed too much) for what they do physically.

The effects can be devastating. No less than 20 to 25 percent of obese children have "hyper-insulinism," that is, they secrete too much insulin—a problem that disappears when they lose weight. High blood pressure can be a problem. And heavy children have more back problems than kids of normal weight. But that's just the beginning.

A study of 538 students in fifth and eighth grades showed that portly kids did more poorly in math and reading than others in their classes. They were "underachievers." According to Anthony Albanese, Ph.D., one of the researchers involved, the children ate too much "low-quality" food, high in calories and low in body-building nutrients. Not only did the heavier children strive less, said Dr. Albanese, but they exhibited "lassitude and irritability" as well.

Researchers agree that obese children may suffer deep emotional disturbances (even if they seem happy on the surface) as a result of being overweight. Some blame all their failures on being fat: the time they weren't asked to the prom, the time they lost the election for class treasurer, and so on. According to Albert Stunkard, M.D., and other experts, parents may subtly encourage their children to maintain an insulation against the world, fearing that a child who becomes attractive to others will also grow less dependent on them.

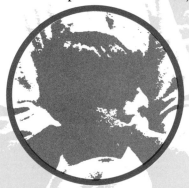

HOW PARENTS CAN HELP

Of course, that's not always the case. Many parents are very concerned about their children's weight problems, but it seems the more they nag, the worse it gets. And trying to enforce a strict diet may have the most damaging results of all: Soon the child is eating "forbidden" foods on the sly and has to cope with feeling guilty and the

---

He's Not Chubby, He's My Child

"I'd say that almost half of all overweight children are not perceived of as overweight by their parents," says Platon Collipp, M.D., head of pediatrics at Nassau County Medical Center, Long Island. "That's because the parents themselves are usually obese, and since that's the way *they* looked as kids, they think their kids look normal. You can't rely on gym teachers to tell parents, either, because they may fear offending them. But if you ask, teachers will tell you where your child stands. Now, a child can be called 'husky' when he's only 10 to 20 percent above ideal body weight; above 20 percent, though, is obese. If a child is obese *and* short in stature, he should see a doctor: diseases that cause obesity can also stunt growth."

fear of being discovered. Eventually, the diet ends in failure. And good riddance, too. Because dieting can be dangerous for a growing child. Children need nutrients to grow and develop properly—*all* the nutrients, including carbohydrates, fats, cholesterol and protein.

But that doesn't mean heavy children shouldn't—and can't—lose weight. Kelly Brownell, Ph.D., believes that children are especially receptive to changing their food habits, even more so than adults, since their eating behavior has had less time to become ingrained. Like other researchers, Dr. Brownell has conducted studies that show behavior modification works well for children. But he also found that parental involvement makes a profound difference in weight loss over the long run—and the *nature* of the participation is critical. In one study with adolescents, he had one group of children attend behavior modification sessions by themselves. Another group attended sessions with their mothers. In the third group, the children attended sessions in one room and the mothers in another. After 16 weeks, the child-alone group lost an average of 7 pounds, the mother-child-together group lost 11½ pounds, and the mother-child-separately group lost 18½ pounds.

Dr. Brownell explains why the mother-child-separately group did so well: "Mothers and children in the mother-child-together group were reluctant to voice negative feelings about the problems of dealing with each other, whereas the mother-child-separately group allowed both parties to discuss sensitive issues."

The best effects, it seems, are achieved when children are allowed to go about changing their eating habits independently, with the support—not the interference—of their parents.

THE PROBLEM CAN BE PREVENTED

Involving parents, therefore, is important in fighting childhood

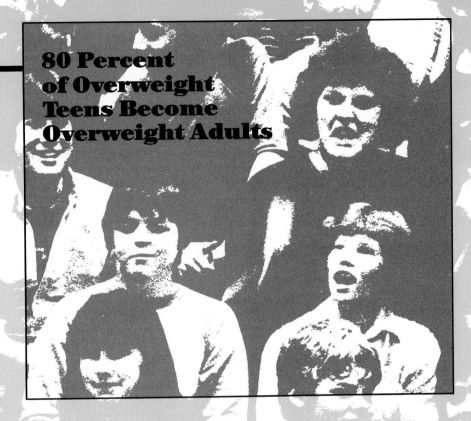

80 Percent of Overweight Teens Become Overweight Adults

obesity. But parents can do a great deal to prevent the problem from happening in the first place.

Rich Binetsky, who endured the pain and ridicule of being a fat child but has lost a great deal of weight as an adult, has strong feelings on the subject. "Pediatricians don't teach us parents the 'right' way to deal with eating, with food and our children," he feels. "Parents need more guidance in this area. You see people all the time giving toddlers something to eat—especially sweet things—to keep them quiet. They are teaching their children to gratify themselves with food, for all situations. Children have no say in this—they can't fend off sweet things flowing their way. If you have to give them food, make it a carrot, at least.

"But it's best not to reward them with food at all," he says. "Give your child a hug, a kiss, a toy, a walk, an outing in the park—some sort of pleasure that's not in the form of food. If parents did that, my guess is that we'd see a drop in adult obesity. It takes a great deal of strength and discipline to do this during those early years, but if you don't want your child to be obese, the easiest way is to establish healthy eating habits from the start."

7

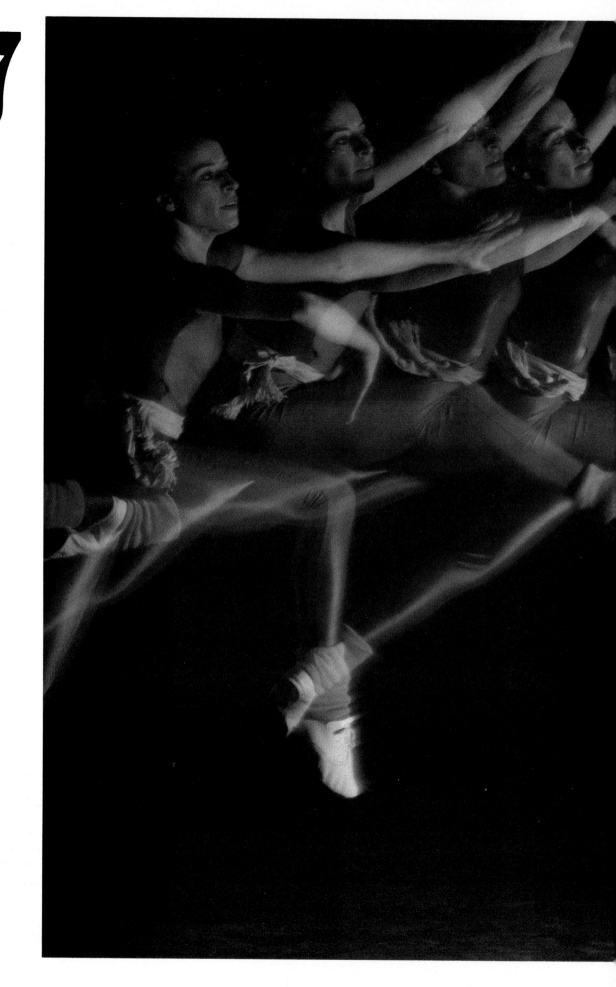

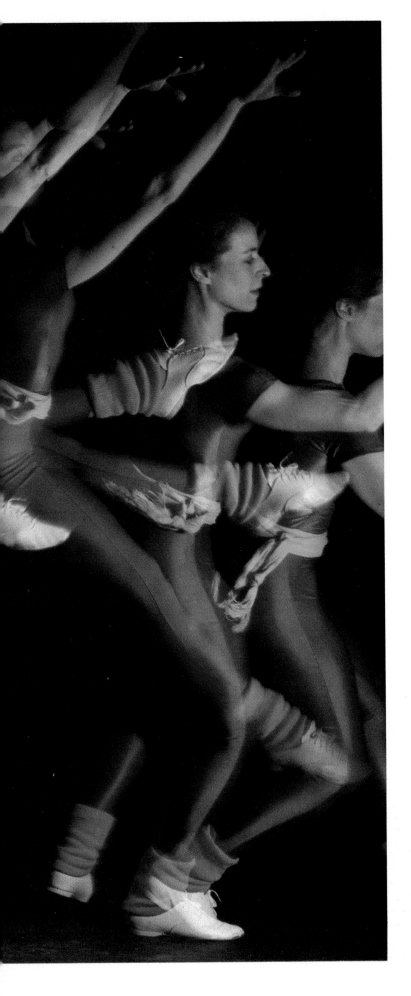

Put Exercise into Your Life

There's no doubt about it. If you want to burn body fat, exercise beats dieting every time.

Without exercise, nearly all attempts to lose weight are doomed to fail. Consider these statistics.

Of all dieters who set out to lose 20 pounds, only 25 percent succeed.

Of those who want to lose 40 pounds, only 5 percent succeed.

And over 90 percent of *all* dieters regain lost pounds within two years.

For all their sacrifices and will power, dieters seem fated to revert to their original weight. And the reason, weight-loss specialists are convinced, is the lack of one key element in their diet regimen: exercise.

Consider the classic case of a group of women who checked into a weight-loss clinic after countless attempts to lose weight. The women were either housewives, teachers, students or receptionists— occupations that, like most jobs today, aren't physically demanding. Over the years, each of the women had lost several pounds by dieting, only to regain the weight again and again.

Doctors at the clinic decided to try a different tack: exercise. They instructed the women to exercise at least 30 minutes a day. All chose walking. And the more the women walked, the more weight they lost, from 10 to 38 pounds the first year. Most important, as long as the women kept walking they never regained any weight. And they did it all without ever changing their eating habits!

So why don't more people exercise?

Hop on the Fat Burner

Certain exercises are just plain better for weight loss because they have the capacity to burn fat while others don't. Aerobic exercises, namely running, rope skipping, brisk walking, aerobic dancing, bicycling, hiking and swimming—anything that gets your heart pumping and your body sweating—are all fat-burning activities.

"What people need is total movement, not head rolls and so forth," emphasizes Barry A. Franklin, Ph.D. "Short, intense activities burn mostly carbohydrates and very little fat. Long-distance activities—and by that I mean walking, swimming, jogging, stationary cycling—burn more fat than carbohydrates." But you do have to pay your dues to garner the reward. Dr. Franklin says it takes 30 minutes of heart-pumping exercise before you are burning fat at peak capacity.

Perhaps it's a matter of misinformation. (We won't accept any other excuse.) Sure, it's true that you'd have to jog for 4 hours just to burn the 3,500 calories equal to 1 pound of fat. And most overweight people could no more run a mile than a marathon. So, they dismiss the idea of exercise altogether.

Yet if you spread that same amount of exercise over the course of a week—and substituted an activity you enjoy, such as dancing, racquetball or walking—you could easily lose a pound a week—without the rigid dietary restrictions.

TRAINING YOUR METABOLISM TO BURN MORE CALORIES

Perhaps the nicest thing about exercise in terms of your weight is the fact that calorie combustion doesn't shut down the minute you kick off your running shoes or jump off your exercise bike. Your body continues to burn extra calories for several hours after you come to rest—even while you sleep! It's sort of like stoking a fire that's about to go out. The few minutes of effort you put into it stirs up enough energy to warm a room all through the night.

Sounds too good to be true, we know. But exercise has the amazing capacity to speed up your metabolism, the rate at which your body burns food and uses energy. Dieting, on the other hand, slows it down. At rest, the unexercised body plods along at an average metabolic rate of about 70 calories an hour. When you cut down on your food consumption through dieting, the metabolic rate slows to about 40 calories per hour—and it stays that way all day long. The reason, explains Gabe Mirkin, M.D., author of *Getting Thin*, is that the body has an adaptive hormone called reverse T_3, which goes into action when calories are reduced. "It's the body's defense against starvation," he says.

However, studies have shown that a dieter who exercises regularly can boost that sluggish rate back to 70 or 80 calories an hour. "Just a half hour a day will keep you burning calories at a faster rate all day long," says Dr. Mirkin.

Another nice thing exercise does for the dieting body is improve its fat-to-muscle ratio. *This ratio is more important than total weight.* The more muscle you have in relation to fat, the more calories you'll burn overall.

"Muscles are little furnaces that avidly metabolize food for energy," says Dr. Mirkin. "Fat storage cells are exactly that—inert depots, for the most part."

Those "inert depots" also take up a lot more room, pound for pound, than muscle. A pound of muscle is not only more active metabolically, it's more densely packed than a pound of fat, so it's smaller. That explains why two women may each weigh 135 pounds, yet one wears a size 10 and the other wears a size 12.

Exercise is the only way you can *build* muscle mass while *decreasing* fat. Studies have shown that those who diet without exercise lose muscle first and fat second.

"With dieting alone, as much as 30 percent of the initial weight loss is muscle," says Ellen Coleman, exercise physiologist and director of the Riverside Cardiac Fitness Center in Riverside, California. "That probably explains why so many dieters look gaunt and saggy—they lose connective tissue along with fat. Exercise, on the other hand, burns fat while increasing muscle tone. So people who exercise to lose weight don't look saggy and wrinkled the way dieters do.

"People need to realize that appearance and percentage of body fat are the *real* measures of weight, not the numbers on their bathroom scales," says Ms. Coleman. "If not, they'll get discouraged and quit exercising. You can lose fat, gain muscle and weigh exactly the same. But you'll look thinner because your percentage of fat will be lower."

EXERCISE REGULATES THE BODY'S FAT BURNERS

If all that weren't enough, exercise has yet another mechanism for burning fat that no other diet method can match. It increases

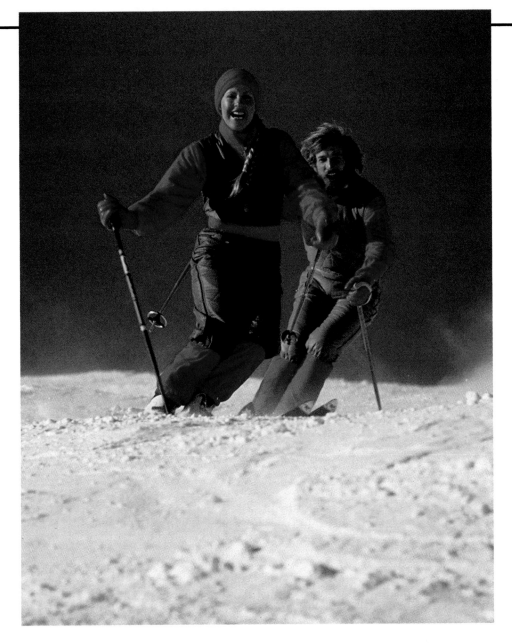

The spray of snow against your body, the warmth of the midday winter sun caressing your face, the exhilaration of streaking down a picturesque mountainside— who says exercise can't be fun! There is no matching a fitness break to keep you in shape and keep your weight down on weekends and vacations. Downhill skiing is just one of the numerous recreational sports that can give you hours of fitness fun.

certain fat-burning enzymes in the muscles—enzymes that gobble fat particles, somewhat like the way Pac Man devours little dots.

"Not only will exercise [build] more muscle, but it will also provide more enzymes to burn the fat," says Dennis Remington, M.D., in his book, *How to Lower Your Fat Thermostat.* "If a person has decreased muscle mass because of dieting, and few enzymes for fat metabolism because of inactivity, the fat particles will simply float around the system for awhile, then return to a fat cell for storage."

Few people realize it, but exercise also controls weight by lowering production of insulin, a hormone that regulates blood sugar.

"Overweight people in general produce four to six times as much insulin as thin people," says Dr. Remington, director of the Eating Disorder Clinic at the Brigham Young University Student Health Center. "And too much insulin prompts the body to convert sugar to fat."

EXERCISE: AN APPETITE SUPPRESSANT

Forget what your instincts tell you. Taking up exercise will not make you hungry.

Take the case of a group of overweight women who were brought into a clinic, ostensibly so researchers could study their metabolic rates. The women did not know the real

(continued on page 110)

Charting Your Progress

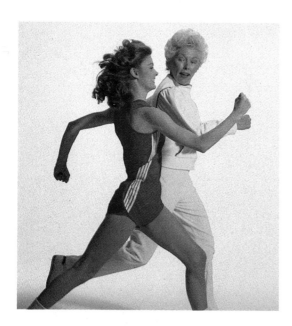

To lose weight, you should strive for an exercise program that burns about 300 calories or more per session. The values given here are approximate for different body weights. In general, though, the more you weigh, the more calories you burn, particularly if you haven't exercised for some time. Overweight or overfat people are less efficient than smaller or more muscular ones—they expend more energy for the same effort. How many calories you burn at each activity will also depend on how intensely you exercise and for how long. For example, a 154-pound person may burn from about 445 to 655 calories in 1 hour of aerobic dance, depending on the intensity of the dancing.

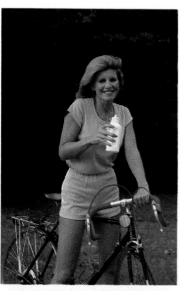

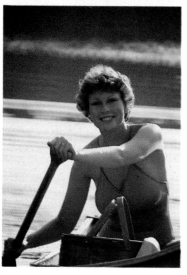

Sports and Other Exercise

Activity	Calories Burned per Hour				
	110 lbs.	132 lbs.	154 lbs.	176 lbs.	198 lbs.
Badminton—singles, recreational	275	310	350	385	425
doubles, recreational	235	270	300	335	365
Basketball—full-court game	585	670	750	830	910
Bicycling—10 mph	325	370	415	460	505
13 mph	515	585	655	725	795
Bowling—regular	150	170	190	210	230
Calisthenics—moderate	350	395	445	490	540
intense	435	495	555	615	675
Canoeing—2 mph	235	270	300	335	365
4 mph	490	560	625	695	765
Dancing—aerobic, moderate	350	395	445	490	540
aerobic, intense	515	585	655	725	795
rock	195	225	250	280	305
square	330	375	420	465	510
waltz	195	225	250	280	305
Football—touch	470	535	600	665	730
Golf—foursome, 9 holes in 2 hrs., pulling clubs	195	225	250	280	305
Handball—2 people	400	455	510	565	620
Hiking—20-lb. pack, 2 mph	235	270	300	335	365
20-lb. pack, 4 mph	355	400	450	500	550
Ice skating	275	310	350	385	425
Martial arts	620	705	790	875	960
Mountain climbing	470	535	600	665	730
Racquetball—2 people	610	695	775	860	945
Roller skating	275	310	350	385	425
Rope skipping—70-80 skips/min.	435	495	555	615	675
90-100 skips/min.	515	585	655	725	795
Rowing—2 mph	235	270	300	335	365
4 mph	515	585	655	725	795
Running—8-min. mile	550	625	700	775	850
Running—12-min. mile	515	585	655	725	795
Running in place—70-80 steps/min.	435	495	555	615	675
90-100 steps/min.	515	585	655	725	795

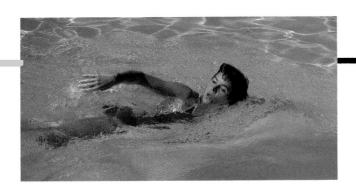

Activity	Calories Burned per Hour				
	110 lbs.	132 lbs.	154 lbs.	176 lbs.	198 lbs.
Scuba diving	355	400	450	500	550
Skiing—cross-country, 5 mph	550	625	700	775	850
downhill	465	530	595	660	720
Soccer	470	535	600	665	730
Swimming—crawl, 30 yards/min.	330	375	420	465	510
crawl, 45 yards/min.	540	615	690	765	835
Stationary bicycle—10 mph	330	375	420	465	515
15 mph	515	585	655	725	795
Tennis—singles, recreational	335	380	425	470	520
doubles, recreational	235	270	300	335	365
Volleyball—recreational	275	310	350	385	425
Walking—2 mph	145	165	185	205	225
3 mph	235	270	300	335	365
5 mph	435	495	555	615	675
Water skiing	375	430	480	535	585
Yoga	180	205	230	255	280

Work and Other Activities

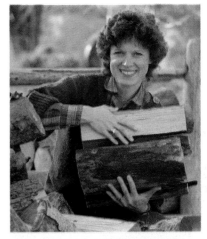

Activity	Calories Burned per Hour				
	110 lbs.	132 lbs.	154 lbs.	176 lbs.	198 lbs.
Bricklaying	160	180	205	225	250
Card playing	70	80	90	100	110
Cooking	105	120	135	150	160
Carpentry—heavy	280	315	355	395	430
light	180	205	230	255	280
Chopping wood—by hand	355	400	450	500	550
with power saw	175	200	220	245	270
Eating	70	80	90	100	110
Farming—with modern machinery	180	205	230	255	280
Gardening	305	345	390	430	470
Housework	160	180	205	225	250
House painting	165	185	210	230	255
Jackhammer—with pneumatic tools	355	400	450	500	550
Lawn mowing—with push mower	360	410	460	510	560
with power mower	195	225	250	280	305
Office work—secretarial	115	130	145	160	175
Raking leaves	175	200	220	245	270
Sawing—by hand	305	350	390	435	475
Sitting, doing handwork	75	85	96	105	115
Sleeping	50	60	65	75	80
Stacking lumber	300	340	380	420	465
Standing	80	90	100	110	120
Stone masonry	300	340	380	420	465
Watching TV	60	70	80	85	95
Washing dishes	105	120	135	150	160
Waiting on tables	190	215	245	270	295
Weeding	235	270	300	335	365
Writing	70	80	90	100	110

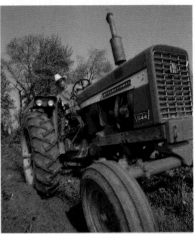

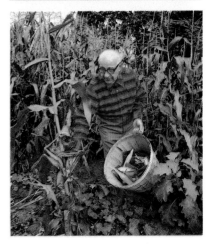

Perhaps the most dramatic way of measuring body fat versus lean body tissue is the underwater submersion test. Through such a test doctors can measure exactly how much fat a person is carrying around. So, who cares? You should, because the ratio of lean body tissue to body fat is what really determines just how good you'll look in the mirror. For women, anything above 22 percent body fat is probably too much. For men, the figure is 19 percent. If you suspect you don't measure up to these figures, there is something you can do about it: exercise.

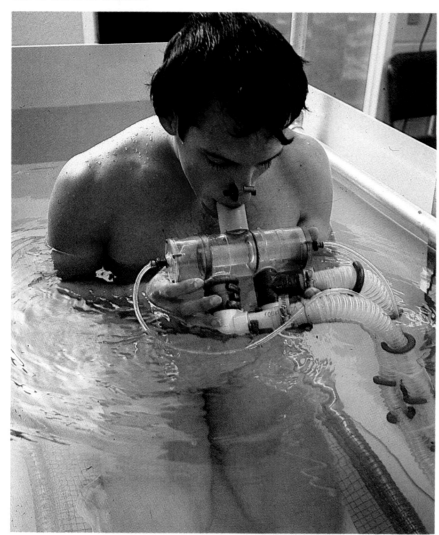

reason for the experiment: to see if exercise would make them hungrier. For the first 19 days, the women were told to follow their customary sedentary habits. They were given all the food they wanted. For the next two 19-day periods, they were put on mild to moderate exercise programs. Again, they were given all the food they wanted, yet they ate no more when they exercised than when they didn't.

"Exercise causes you to burn more calories on the one hand and to eat less on the other," says Dr. Mirkin. "This way, it satisfies both sides of the weight-loss equation."

GIVE YOUR MOOD A BOOST

Besides burning fat and calories directly, exercise helps you slim down in other, less direct ways.

First off, exercise recharges your mental batteries. Anyone who's been on a crash diet knows that it can leave you tired, cranky and apathetic. But exercise does just the opposite. And that's not a pep talk, it's a fact: When you exercise, your body releases noradrenaline, a hormone that works on your brain to help change frowns into smiles.

Second, a workout can reduce stress and tension—and that means you're less likely to use food as an antistress tranquilizer.

"One of the best ways to cope with stress is to exercise," says Dr. Remington. "If you find yourself tense or angry, take a brisk walk, chop wood or play a hard game of racquetball." So next time you feel boxed in or uptight, reach for sneakers instead of a snack!

A WHOLE-BODY APPROACH TO EXERCISE

If you think exercise begins and ends with jogging, you're in for some pleasant surprises. While jogging may be fine for some people, there are plenty of other options from which to choose.

"If you don't like to jog, try walking," says Dr. Bernard Gutin, of Columbia. "If swimming isn't your cup of tea, try bicycling. There are enough choices available to ensure that you'll find something you enjoy."

But whatever activity you choose—walking, bicycling, swimming, jogging—it has to be *aerobic*. That means you do it for 20 or 30 minutes at least three times a week, and keep the pace brisk enough so that your heart pumps hard. That type of exercise forces you to use large amounts of oxygen, to really *breathe*. And anything that burns a lot of oxygen also burns a lot of fat and calories.

Exercises such as calisthenics and weight training are *anaerobic*. They demand brief spurts of intense effort—enough to draw a bead or two of sweat, but not enough to burn a lot of calories. That doesn't mean anaerobic activities are useless, though. They're excellent for flexing, toning and firming muscles. The ideal program of exercise for weight loss should include both.

EXERCISE A LA CARTE

You should choose the type of exercise you will enjoy and stick with. However, keep in mind that some activities are more practical and effective than others. Here's a rundown on some of the most popular aerobic activities and their value in weight loss.

Walking. "The great advantage of walking is that it can be done anywhere, by anyone, regardless of age or sex," says Kenneth Cooper, M.D., the "father of aerobics" and author of *The Aerobics Program for Total Well-Being.* Other doctors agree.

"If you are extremely overweight, walking is your wisest choice," says Bud Getchell, Ph.D., founder of the human performance laboratory at Ball State University, Muncie, Indiana. Dr. Getchell recommends that people begin by walking less than a mile at a stretch, building up to 2 miles, then 3 or 4, until they can walk 3 to 3½ miles in 45 to 60 minutes. And it works! Remember, the women we discussed in the beginning of this chapter did nothing more than add a daily walk to their schedule.

Running or Jogging. Walking is roughly defined as a pace that covers about 1 mile in 14 minutes or more. Cover the same distance in 8 to 12 minutes and you're running.

The advantage to running is that it's more intense, so you burn more calories while running than while walking for the same amount of time. If you walk for 10 minutes, you'll burn 35 calories. If you run for 10 minutes, you'll burn 141—more than four times as much.

"Almost anyone who gets into running and stays with it loses weight," says Dr. Mirkin in his book. "The more miles you run, and the faster you run them, the trimmer you get, no matter how much you eat."

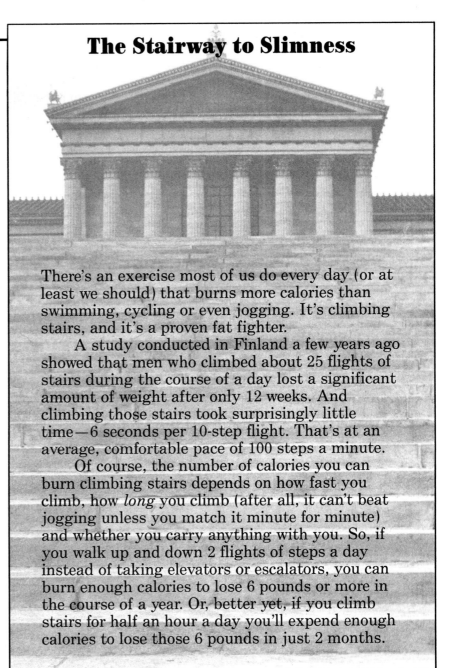

The Stairway to Slimness

There's an exercise most of us do every day (or at least we should) that burns more calories than swimming, cycling or even jogging. It's climbing stairs, and it's a proven fat fighter.

A study conducted in Finland a few years ago showed that men who climbed about 25 flights of stairs during the course of a day lost a significant amount of weight after only 12 weeks. And climbing those stairs took surprisingly little time—6 seconds per 10-step flight. That's at an average, comfortable pace of 100 steps a minute.

Of course, the number of calories you can burn climbing stairs depends on how fast you climb, how *long* you climb (after all, it can't beat jogging unless you match it minute for minute) and whether you carry anything with you. So, if you walk up and down 2 flights of steps a day instead of taking elevators or escalators, you can burn enough calories to lose 6 pounds or more in the course of a year. Or, better yet, if you climb stairs for half an hour a day you'll expend enough calories to lose those 6 pounds in just 2 months.

Swimming and Aqua Aerobics. Water exercises are excellent for overweight people because water supports the body. You don't subject your bones, joints and muscles to the beating they can get on a running track, yet you can still burn enough fat and calories to help you shed pounds.

Swimming laps isn't the only aerobic water exercise. Aqua aerobics are to swimming what aerobic dancing is to ballet—without muscle soreness. Aqua aerobics consists of activities such as scissor kicks, leg lifts and "sprints" through the water—giving you a good workout with nary a callus in the process.

(continued on page 114)

Fitness at the Starting Line

If it's been years since you did anything more strenuous than walk the dog, you can't expect to run out the door and start exercising like an Olympic contender. Start slow and easy to prevent soreness and injury.

1. Relaxation. Lie on the floor with knees bent and arms outstretched. Take several long, slow, deep breaths. Clench your fists for 2 or 3 seconds and release.

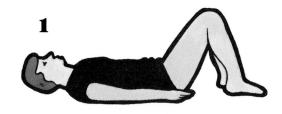

2. Lower Back and Hip Stretcher. Lie on your back with knees straight. Pull one knee to your chest. Grasp the leg just below the knee and pull the knee toward your chest. Hold for 5 seconds, then curl your head and shoulders toward the knee. Hold 5 seconds longer. Repeat the exercise with the other leg. Exercise each leg 4 times.

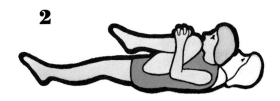

3. Leg Stretcher. Lie on your back with knees bent. Slowly bring one knee to your chest, then slowly straighten your leg until it's at a 45- to 90-degree angle. Hold for 8 to 10 seconds. Keep your leg straight while you lower it to the floor, and then return to a bent-knee position. Repeat with the other leg.

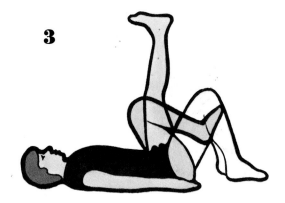

Before You Begin

- Get a "green light" from your doctor, particularly if you're over 35 or have heart, back or other health problems. You may be asked to take an EKG test (to measure heart rhythm) or a stress test (to measure heart and lung health).
- Choose "soft" exercises, such as swimming, aqua aerobics, walking or cycling. They're kind to rusty joints.
- Make a concerted effort to go *slowly*. You should work up a sweat, but don't overexert yourself. During a workout, you should be able to converse comfortably. If you can't, ease off. And stop if you feel pain.

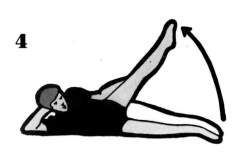

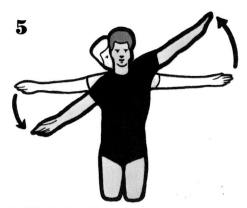

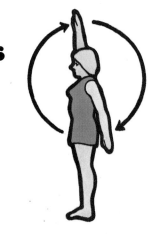

4. Side Leg Raises. Lie on your side with your head resting on your hand and your feet together. Raise your upper leg from the floor, keeping it straight with the toes pointed. Lower to starting position. Alternate sides and repeat 10 times with each leg.

5. Windmills. Kneel, keeping your waist and back straight. With arms outstretched to the sides, lean to one side. Place your lower hand as close to the floor as possible while raising your other hand. Return to starting position and lean to the other side. Repeat 8 times on each side.

6. Arm Circles. Stand with your feet shoulder-width apart. Swing your arms forward, making large sweeping circles. Repeat 10 times, then reverse the swing and repeat 10 more times.

7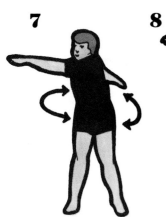

8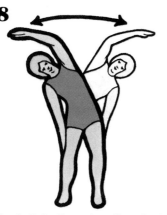

9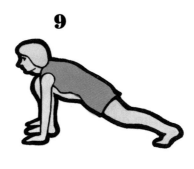

10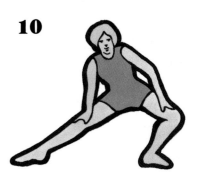

7. Trunk Twister. Stand with your feet shoulder-width apart, arms extended to the sides at shoulder level. Keeping your heels on the floor, slowly twist your torso to one side as far as you can. Return to starting position, then twist slowly to the other side. Repeat for a total of 6 complete twists.

8. Side Stretcher. Stand with your feet shoulder-width apart, with one arm extended upward (palm facing inward) and the other arm extended downward (palm touching the outside of your thigh). Lean to that side, sliding your hand down your leg as far as you can comfortably reach. Switch arms and repeat on the other side. Do this stretch 6 times on each side.

9. Forward Lunge. With your palms on the floor, move one foot forward so that it is flexed under your chest and your knee is directly over the ankle. Stretch your other leg out behind you. Roll your body forward while pushing your hips toward the floor. *Don't bounce.* Hold for 5 seconds or longer. Reverse legs and repeat. Stretch each leg 5 times.

11. Wall Pushups. Stand 3 feet from a wall, facing it. With hands resting on the wall, lean forward, bending your elbows slowly. With legs and torso straight, lean closer to the wall, without lifting your feet or heels off the floor. Hold for 10 seconds. Repeat with knees bent.

10. Side Lunge. Spread your legs in a wide straddle position, toes pointing straight ahead. Shift your weight to one side so that most of your weight is on one leg. *Don't bounce.* Hold this position for 5 seconds or longer. Shift your weight to the other leg and repeat. Repeat 4 times on each side.

11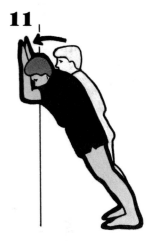

12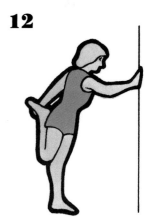

12. Standing Quad Stretcher. Stand erect and balance yourself with your hand against a wall or chair. Bend one knee and draw the leg up and back. Hold. Pull your foot gently until you feel slight discomfort in the upper front thigh. Hold for 5 seconds or longer. Repeat with the other leg.

Before Each Workout

Cold, stiff muscles and tendons are never ready to spring immediately into action, no matter how in shape you are. You must warm and stretch muscles and get your blood moving before you start *any* vigorous activity.

- Begin warming up by doing the simple relaxation technique shown in Figure 1. Then work into your activity gradually. If you're going to run or jog, walk slowly for 5 to 10 minutes. If you're going to cycle, cycle slowly at first. A gradual start also stimulates the heart and lungs.

- If your back and shoulder muscles feel tight, do the stretches shown in Figures 2, 3 and 4. If your arm and back muscles feel stiff, do stretches 5, 6, 7 and 8. If your leg or calf muscles feel tight, do stretches 9, 10, 11 and 12. Always stretch any muscle that's ever given you trouble in the past.

After Each Workout

When you're finished working out, don't stop abruptly and dash for the shower. Cooling your muscles is just as important as warming them up.

- Keep moving for another 5 to 10 minutes, tapering off gradually. Walking is the easiest way to cool down—it helps your muscles pump blood from your arms and legs back to the heart and brain and allows your heart rate and blood pressure to return to normal.

- To complete the cool-down phase, do all of the stretching and relaxation exercises in Figures 1 through 12, *in reverse order.* This will prevent your muscles from locking into a contraction or spasms, so they will be limber, not stiff, the next day. In fact, the more you stretch *after* each workout, the less you'll need to stretch before your next session.

Walk, Don't Rest, after Meals

After a big meal, your body whispers "Move, take a walk!" As usual, your body's right. Researchers have found that even moderate exercise an hour or so after eating helps you more efficiently burn the calories that might otherwise have wrapped around your waist.

In a study at Cornell University, David Levitsky, Ph.D., an associate professor of nutrition, found that when volunteers ate normally and then walked briskly for 20 minutes the next day, their bodies burned off 10 to 15 percent more calories than they did without the walk. But when the subjects overate, then walked briskly the next day, their bodies burned off almost *50 percent* of the calories. He suggests a 20-minute walk 1 to 3 hours after a meal.

To get the most out of aqua aerobics, you can attach inflatable cuffs, called floats, to your wrists and ankles. The water pushes up on the light, air-filled sacs, coaxing you to work your arms and legs a little bit harder.

Cycling. On the road or on a stationary bike, cycling is a good choice for overweight people because it's easy on the legs yet still burns enough oxygen to qualify as aerobic. And for people who are "too busy to exercise" or who consider themselves unathletic, stationary cycling has a real edge over road cycling: You can cycle in the privacy of your own home, whenever you feel like it, at your own pace.

Aerobic Dancing. Basically, aerobic dancing is a program of various exercises set to music. It includes walking, running, hopping, skipping and various kicks and arm swings, plus a few calisthenics thrown in for variety.

Aerobic dance classes consist of groups of women *and* men, plus a leader. Once you learn a few routines, you can work out at home to aerobic programs on TV, tapes or records. Be sure to move every part of the body in the course of your at-home routine—arms, legs, torso and so forth. And move quickly from one set of exercises to the next, to reap the full benefit of this popular fat-burning activity.

Rope Skipping. This is another convenient, inexpensive aid to weight loss. Dr. Cooper recommends that you wear athletic shoes and skip on a cushioned surface such as a thick carpet. Do it to music, to make it more entertaining. And don't do too much, too soon. Warm up first by skipping slowly or walking briskly for 3 minutes. Begin with six 20-second sessions with 10-second intervals between them. Gradually work up to a point where you can skip for 10 minutes at a time.

Mini-Trampolines or Rebounders. Early research suggested that mini-trampolines (called rebounders) provided aerobic exercise. But more recent studies say that you really have to jump with all your heart for trampolines to do any good.

"Mini-trampolines do not burn a lot of calories, because the machine does some work for you by pushing you back upward," says Barry A. Franklin, Ph.D., director of the cardiac rehabilitation program at Sinai Hospital of Detroit, Michigan. "They might be a good way to begin if you've never exercised or if you have orthopedic problems. But for real weight loss, I recommend activities that involve total body movement in which the participant supplies the energy."

Court Sports: Racquetball, Tennis, Handball and Squash. We lump these activities together because they all provide about the same type and amount of exercise. Yet there are subtle differences. One advantage of racquetball, for instance, is that it's easier to learn than tennis. Also, with four walls and a ceiling to hit and no net to block your shots, there's more action.

"Still, you have to be quite skilled at racquetball to keep moving for the 30 minutes or so necessary to burn fat," says Ms. Coleman. "And you have to be in fairly good shape to begin with."

The same could be said for most court sports. Thus, people who are new to exercise are generally better off beginning with easier exercises and adding court sports later, if they wish.

Cross-Country Skiing. Also called Nordic skiing, cross-country skiing can add spice to your exercise routine if you live in a snowy area. Simply walk your skis across the fields and hills, mapped trails, parks or golf courses. Olympic-caliber skiers can burn up to 1,000 calories an hour, but even a beginner can burn quite a bit of fat and calories on the trail. Anyone can do it, and by the second try it will seem quite natural. Besides, there's all that snow to catch you if you fall, leaving only your dignity bruised.

HOW MUCH? HOW OFTEN?

If you choose the right form of exercise, you may begin to see results in as little as four weeks, says Ms. Coleman. If you don't, ask yourself these questions.

Are you eating more and not admitting it? As we said before, exercise shouldn't increase your appetite. In some cases, though, people use exercise as an excuse to overeat. True, exercise allows you to get away with a certain amount of minor "cheating." But if you go overboard, you can still end up eating more calories than you burn off. For example, if you treat yourself to a large pizza and a few beers after every workout, you can't expect to lose weight. For best results, you should couple exercise with caloric vigilance. Exercise and dieting are better than either one alone.

Are you working hard enough? "You have to do enough work to burn at least 300 calories or more per session," says Ms. Coleman. "That's roughly equal to walking or jogging 3 miles, bicycling 12 miles or swimming 1 mile."

If that sounds like more than you can handle, the researchers we spoke to suggested combining activities.

"Skip rope for 10 minutes, walk for 10, then dance for 10—whatever arrangement you like," says Ms. Coleman. "As long as it's continuous."

Continuous? Won't I get pooped?

"I advise people to start slowly and build up, then ease back—staying within 60 to 80 percent of their maximum heart rate," says Ms. Coleman.

Maximum heart rate is the algebra of health: Subtract your age from 220, then calculate 60 to 80 percent of that figure. If you're 40 years old, for instance, your pulse rate during exercise should range from 60 percent of 180 (108 beats per minute) to 80 percent of 180 (144 beats per minute). Anything lower than that means you're not working hard enough. Anything higher means you should slow down.

Are you exercising often enough? No matter how earnestly you exercise, it won't do any good if your workouts are few and far between.

"People need to exercise a minimum of three times a week," says Dr. Franklin. "Exercising twice a week is not sufficient to lose weight."

The hardest part about exercise is getting started, the experts say. But once you get going, you'll find it well worth your while. As Dr. Remington puts it:

"Exercise is a lot like knitting a sweater. If each stitch is viewed as the total product, it seems tedious. But by visualizing each stitch as a step toward finishing a beautiful sweater, you remain interested in the work and find great satisfaction as the sweater takes shape—until at last you have something you can be proud of."

So tough it out. Each lap across the pool, turn around the track, or mile on your bike will take you closer to having a body you can be proud of!

Body Wraps: Bound for Weight Loss?

Want to lose a few fast pounds in a few short hours? Or whittle away inches with no effort at all?

That sounds too good to be true—and it is. Advertisements for body wraps claim all you need do is lather your body with some "special" cream and wrap yourself up in cellophane (or other nonporous material) and presto—in less than an hour you're slimmer and trimmer. And it's true. In less than an hour you are slimmer and trimmer—but only for about another hour or so. After a few glasses of water your weight will be right back where it started. Because it's only water, *not* fat, that you shed in the body wrap.

As for the inches, well, they'll bounce back, too. For instance, if you twist a rubber band around your finger, leave it there and remove it a few minutes later, you'll have an indentation on your finger—a temporary one. The same thing happens if you wrap your body tightly in something—whether it be cellophane or a girdle. The inches aren't lost, merely shifted. They'll creep back to normal in a matter of time.

So the answer's no. You're not bound for weight loss in a body wrap. Only disappointment.

The Spa Treatment

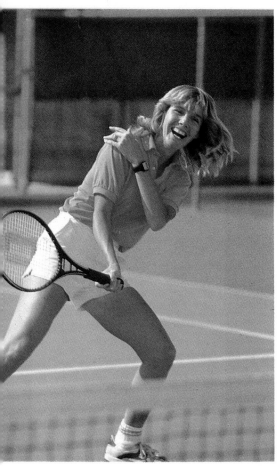

Take up exercise. Avoid temptation. Give up binge food—forever. It all sounds so simple in theory. But when it comes down to real-life practice, we all know how hard it really can be. There are overtime work schedules to meet, children to feed, a skinny spouse snacking on ice cream and that dinner party coming up Saturday night. No wonder your diet isn't getting you anywhere. It's not always your fault!

Wouldn't it be nice if you could get away from it all to some weight watcher's paradise—a place where diet meals taste like they came from gourmet restaurants, where the urge to exercise comes as often as the urge to eat and inches melt away like butter under the midday sun.

Wishful thinking? It doesn't have to be. We found such a place tucked in the foothills of the majestic Santa Catalina Mountains near Tucson, Arizona. It's the Canyon Ranch Spa, a vacation resort dedicated to getting its guests fit and trim. What's it like spending a week at a spa? Well, turn the page and you'll find out.

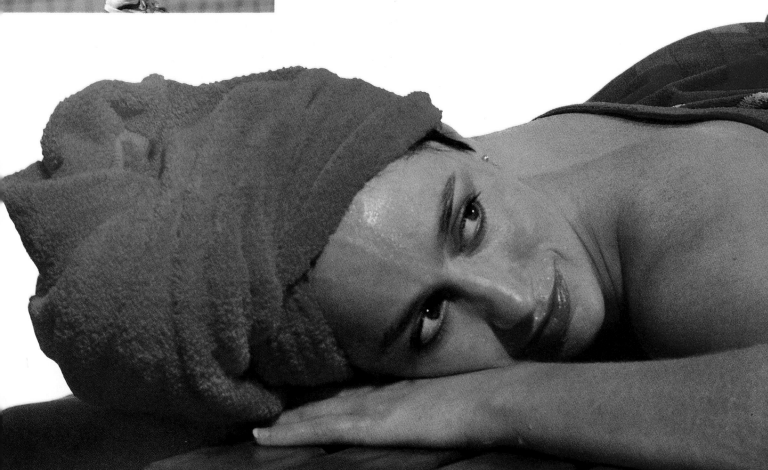

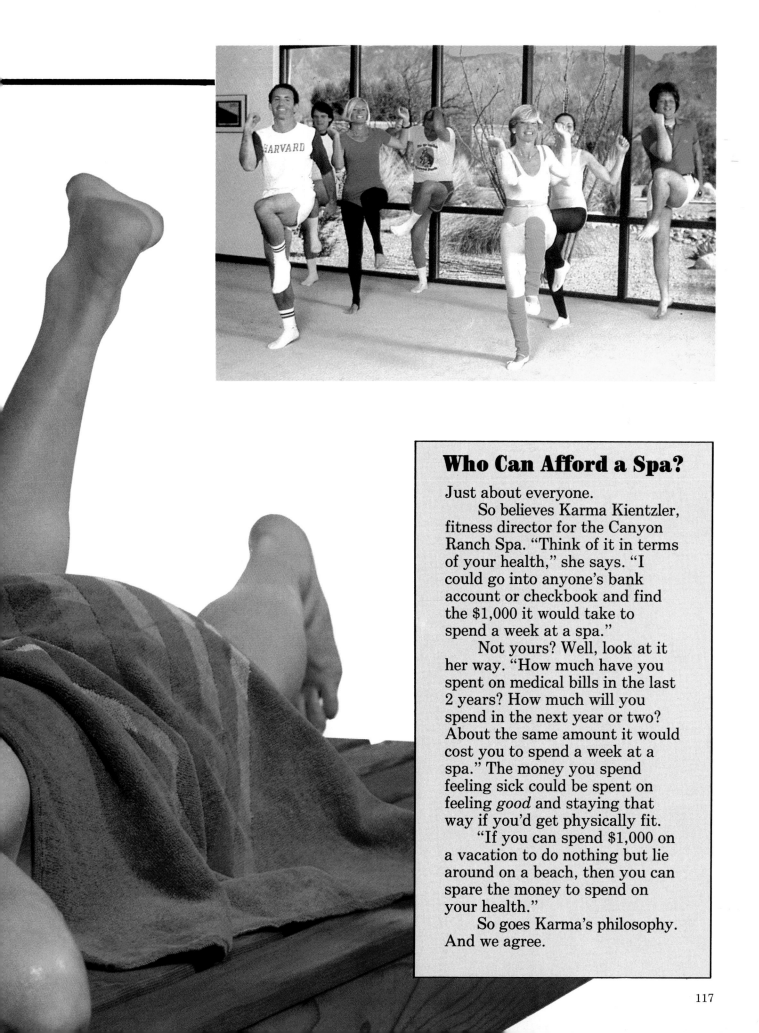

Who Can Afford a Spa?

Just about everyone.

So believes Karma Kientzler, fitness director for the Canyon Ranch Spa. "Think of it in terms of your health," she says. "I could go into anyone's bank account or checkbook and find the $1,000 it would take to spend a week at a spa."

Not yours? Well, look at it her way. "How much have you spent on medical bills in the last 2 years? How much will you spend in the next year or two? About the same amount it would cost you to spend a week at a spa." The money you spend feeling sick could be spent on feeling *good* and staying that way if you'd get physically fit.

"If you can spend $1,000 on a vacation to do nothing but lie around on a beach, then you can spare the money to spend on your health."

So goes Karma's philosophy. And we agree.

"How long are you in for?" quips Jerry to another "newcomer" as they wait for a fitness consultation shortly after their arrival "on the ranch."

"Ten days," comes the reply from the young woman, who hastily adds she hopes to shed 10 pounds and just as many inches in so many days.

"I'm in for 30 days," smiles Jerry as he nervously taps his well-stretched red and white polo shirt. His protruding stomach makes his midsection somewhat resemble a beach ball. It makes the young woman smile. "Take lots of hikes. The hikes are great around here," Jerry advises her. "They're a real workout. They'll help you take it off."

The conversation is cut short by the presence of Randy Raugh, a member of Canyon Ranch's knowledgeable and dedicated fitness staff. "Who's first?" he asks the fit and not-so-fit standing before him. "Me," pipes up Jerry and they soon are huddled in conversation over the long list of activities this fitness kingdom has to offer.

There's no doubt about it. Fitness is serious business at Canyon Ranch and everyone is coached on the proper program to follow *before* they ever set a sneaker onto a gym floor. And fitness director Karma Kientzler has made sure there are plenty of fitness opportunities available to suit anyone's ability. She takes pride in the fact that anyone from the most out-of-shape, overweight sloth to a triathlon master can all walk away from a Karma Kientzler-designed fitness program feeling renewed.

But most of the people who go to Canyon Ranch are on a fitness level somewhere in between—like Jerry and his new-found fitness friend. With Randy's advice and fitness information in tow, the two set out for the warm Arizona sunshine raring to dive into their self-improvement adventure. "Now go to the nurse to get weighed and checked out, then spend the afternoon going to some of the classes, if you like. You can get into the full

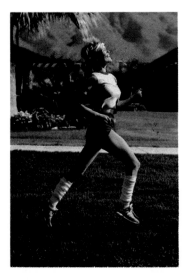

swing of it tomorrow, starting with the morning walk," he says.

Of course, Randy fails to mention that the morning walk begins before the night ends for most people. As alarm clocks buzz at a sleepy 6 A.M. in the late January chill, darkness still fills the sky and frost is nipping the tall and imposing saguaro cacti which spot the desert scenery. No one *makes* you get up so early at Canyon Ranch (after all, it is a vacation resort). Yet, just about everybody does. Just one day out in the desert dawn is enough to convince even the most inert guests that an invigorating walk is a great way to start the day. (But there is a pecuniary motivation, too. The fact that you're paying anywhere from $1,000 to $1,500 per week for the experience makes it only prudent to participate.)

On this particular Monday morning they stand in the morning freshness, a hundred or so strong. Men, but mostly women. Young to old. Lean to not so lean.

Randy is standing at the head of the pack. "We'll start by warming up," he says. "Warming up is very important." Everyone stretches, slowly and easily.

"See that house up there?" he says now, quite serious, pointing to a white stucco adobe perched near the crest of a steep hill. "That's where the 4-miler goes. The going is rough and we go at a pretty good clip." And the walk begins—with most people opting *not* to follow Randy today.

"This is an aerobic workout," coaches Robin, one of the spa's many pretty and trim fitness leaders, to those who stay behind. "We will be taking a 2-mile walk and will go at a pace to give you heart-pumping exercise." And off they go. Robin is in the lead and another staffer is on the tail. It's another amenity of the spa's smartly crafted exercise program. The byword is always "go at your own pace" and there's always a person at the front and the back of a group—whether it's the morning walk or a grueling mountain hike—to make the easygoing feel at ease. As the sun comes

A Spa Meal

During a 10-day stay at the Canyon Ranch Spa guests have the opportunity to experience the 30 different meals Jeanne Jones, author and health food expert, devised for the spa. The meal at right is Shades of Green Salad, Shrimp Curry with Chutney, Brown Rice and Pineapple Boat with Coconut Sauce. Total calories: 373.

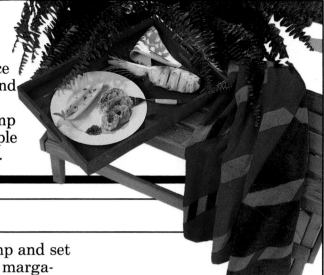

Shrimp Curry

Makes 4 servings

2 cups medium shrimp
1½ teaspoons corn oil margarine
2 small onions, minced
2½ tablespoons whole wheat flour
2 teaspoons curry powder
⅛ teaspoon ground ginger
½ cup chicken stock
1½ cups skim milk, warmed

Clean the shrimp and set aside. Melt the margarine in a 4½-quart pot. Add the onions and cook, covered, until clear and tender, 3 to 5 minutes.

Combine the flour, curry powder and ginger in a small bowl. Add the flour mixture to the onions, stirring constantly, until it forms a thick paste. Add the stock and stir again.

Slowly add the warm milk, stirring constantly.

Cook slowly over low heat, stirring frequently, until the sauce thickens slightly, about 15 minutes. Add the shrimp and heat thoroughly, about 5 minutes. Do not overcook shrimp.

Serve over brown rice.

---

up they wind through the desert streets, slightly uphill and slightly down. Nothing too hard, but hard enough to make many lose pace with the leader. When they return a half hour later, the sun is shining and warm and the smell of breakfast is in the air. They oblige the leader's plea to partake of a few important minutes of cool-down exercise. But many eyes are fixed on the dining room door. For at Canyon Ranch, mealtime is taken just as seriously as exercise.

The reason is more than mere hunger after a healthy morning walk. Everyone finds the food at Canyon Ranch genuinely delicious. Besides, at the suggested 800 calories per day for women and 1,000 calories for men, no one dares miss a meal. Of course, no one is *made* to keep within such restrictions. Seconds and even thirds are yours for the asking. Yet, the same urge that compels you to want to exercise

finds you compulsively counting your calories, too. Jeanne Jones, the gourmet food expert who designed the menu, has carte blanche from spa owners Mel and Enid Zuckerman to use all the imagination and extravagance necessary to make eating the Canyon Ranch way a unique experience. But the uniqueness goes beyond the use of truffles, fine cheeses and the freshest of fruits and vegetables from around the world in the recipes. Canyon Ranch also bars salt, sugar and alcohol from the tables, and caffeine from the coffee and tea. The guests are put on a diet low in saturated fats and high in fiber. The diet is 80 percent complex carbohydrates—lots of grains, fruits and vegetables. Only 4 ounces of protein—and that, of course, includes any meats and cheese—are put into the 800-calorie menu. Complaints? Hardly ever. Even the meat-and-potatoes crowd find it a refreshing change.

With all these restrictions, breakfast, obviously, is quite different from the fare you find at home. This morning's suggestion is listed on the board: breakfast pizza with fresh fruit at a mere 172 calories. It's a piece of whole wheat English muffin heaped with a strawberry topping and low-fat cheese. But there is also freshly squeezed orange juice, succulent grapefruit, the ever-popular Canyon Ranch bread (at 45 calories a slice) and a variety of daily cereals. Oh, yes, and there's the morning multiple vitamin, approved by the registered dietitian on the staff.

Resort to Fitness

With some 80 spas scattered throughout the country, it only makes sense to do a little shopping before committing your bulges and budget to a program of self-improvement.

If money is a problem, you'll be happy to know there are several good spas in the "modest" range of $400 to $500 a week, such as The Oaks in Ojai, California, or the Carmel Country Spa in northern California.

Also, you'll want to make sure the place you choose is dedicated to fitness and weight loss. If you're not a self-starter, a spa with a do-your-own-thing attitude may not be for you. Also, some, like the Main Chance in Phoenix, Arizona, emphasize beauty rather than fitness. Others are nothing more than posh country clubs for the super rich. (We know of one where the guests don't even get out of bed until noon!)

How are you supposed to find all this out? Send for brochures and comb newspapers and magazines for stories on spas. When you narrow your choices down to a few, call the director of each one. Ask about staff credentials, staff-to-guest ratio and if the diet is supervised by a registered dietitian.

If possible, talk to people who have been there. They'll be able to tell you better than anybody what to expect. *The Spa Book,* by Judy Babcock and Judy Kennedy, is also a good reference.

The dining room, which overlooks mesquite trees and is lighted by an enormous skylight, has the ambience to keep people lingering over their decaf until the 9 A.M. classes are ready to begin. Some of the men head off to a stretch class scheduled for males only. For others it's the tennis courts or jogging trails. But the most popular class at this time on this day seems to be something called Stretch and Flex, a class, the brochure says, designed to "enhance muscle tone, increase flexibility and prevent sore muscles." Robin Bortnick, petite, pretty and the essence of the proverbial body beautiful in her shimmering tights and leotard, eases the classes into rhythmic motion to the soothing voice of Linda Ronstadt. Robin whispers above the recording, so as not to spoil the cadence. "Stretch, 1-2-3-4. Flex, 2-3-4." Arms rotate until they feel they will break. You "lift left leg and hold, 1-2. And right, 3-4" until you can't any longer. Ten minutes pass. Twenty minutes pass. Isn't this ever going to end? Forty-five minutes pass. You stop. Ah, you find you're feeling wonderful!

Ten o'clock finds you moving to a second class—Fitness First, another dose of what you just went through but with a brief aerobic interlude. Instead of Ronstadt, you have the fast pace of Barbra Streisand. "Run forward, kick. Back, 1-2, kick. Get those bods moving!" comes the voice of willowy Dee Trayers. Some gasp for breath. Others are only revving up. After this class, you tell yourself, you'll take a breather and relax by the pool. But somehow, come 11 A.M., that invisible arm is behind you, prodding you off to yet another class. Oh, where are you getting the energy! You head for the killer class they call Positive Power.

Positive Power is not easy and definitely not for the new or even the not-so-new to exercise. It is stretching. It is moving. It is heart and muscle pushed to the breaking point and then pushed even more. It's 75 minutes of grueling exercise warmed up to through stretches you never dreamed existed. "R-e-a-c-h!"

bellows Karma as the class, some 20 strong, sweep about the floor. "Kick!" Karma's shocking pink jumpsuit rolls through the movements as naturally as waves come in from the sea. Fifty minutes pass. Some people sneak out the door, huffing. Sixty minutes pass. Another few drop out. But Karma's still at it and so is the healthy group behind her.

It's now 12:15 and the dining room is already full. What will it be for lunch today? A marinated vegetable salad, a fresh, juicy baked tomato and crepes florentine—just one—for a total of 207 calories. Yes, there's one other thing you learn quickly at Canyon Ranch. *Good* food does not mean *lots* of food.

You linger once again over your decaf. Afternoon exercise doesn't start for another hour. But what should you do? There are more classes in the gym, including one especially to help shape up the body; there are workouts in the pool, circuit training on the spa's sophisticated body-contouring machinery, hikes, swimming, biking, tennis, yoga, racquetball. And, of course, you can't leave without the pleasurable pursuits—pedicures, manicures, facials, full-body massages, herbal wraps, plus sauna, steam bath, Jacuzzi, eucalyptus room and sunbathing au naturel.

You opt for a bike ride this afternoon, a facial and massage tonight, a hike tomorrow afternoon and a massage and pedicure tomorrow night.

A while later, after your dinner of salad, shrimp curry with chutney (there are but 4 shrimp) and pineapple with coconut sauce and brown rice—a grand total of 373 calories—comes the soothing warmth of hands and feet being tucked into warm little mittens before the evening's facial treatment. Ah, you tell yourself, you really deserve this. A massage afterward and you barely find the energy to fall into bed.

But the next morning, the zest to try it all again appears with the 6 o'clock alarm. You're warming up for the morning walk—this time the 4-miler. You're stretching and

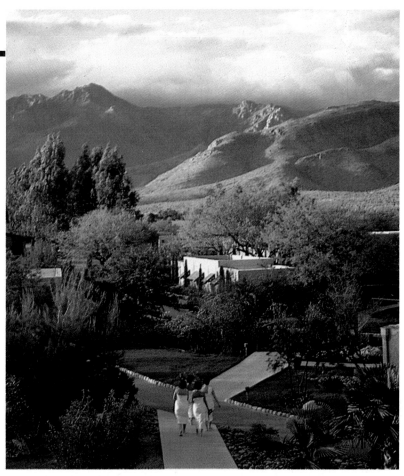

As the sun sets over the majestic Santa Catalina Mountains near Tucson, Arizona, spa-goers head for a relaxing massage at the Canyon Ranch Spa.

flexing, perspiring through Positive Power. Your muscles ache. You vow to stop—to take the day off—but that mysterious urge has you going from one class to another—3 hours of classes in the morning, tennis in the afternoon, jogging in the evening before dinner. You're glowing with pleasure at your accomplishment.

By the third day, the aches and pains are gone, your waistline feels thinner, there is a warm, healthy glow about your face.

Is it really possible to leave inches and pounds behind in just 1 week at a spa? "If you work at it, the answer is yes," says Karma.

But the key to keeping it off is continuing the same diligent work after you leave a spa. Karma knows that all too well. After all, she gets to meet a lot of people at Canyon Ranch—some time and again. Like Jerry. Can he really lose 30 pounds in his 30-day stay? "Oh, sure," he says with much confidence. "I did it before and I can do it again. But this time"—he pauses—"I intend it to be the last."

8

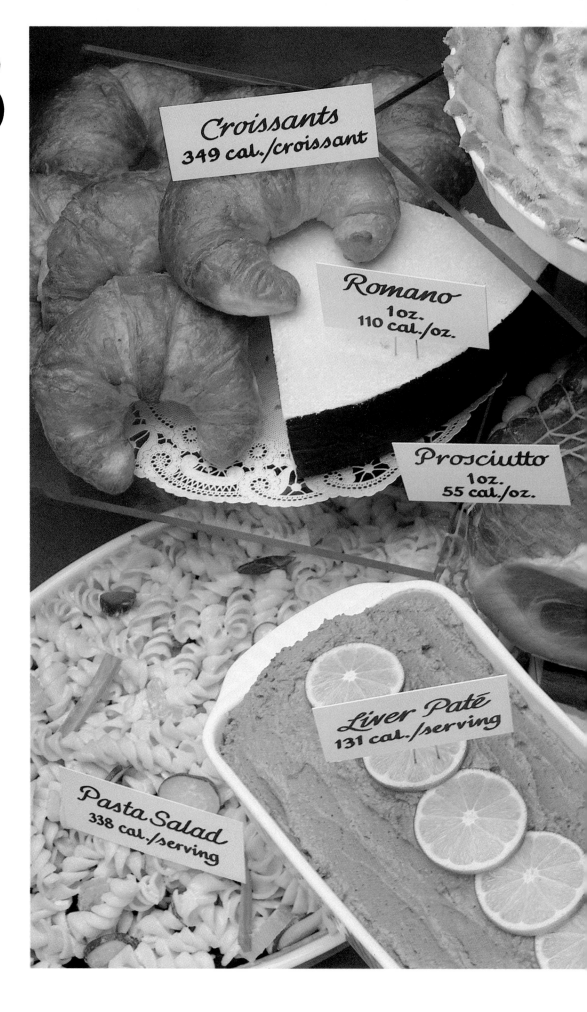

Croissants
349 cal./croissant

Romano
1oz.
110 cal./oz.

Prosciutto
1oz.
55 cal./oz.

Liver Paté
131 cal./serving

Pasta Salad
338 cal./serving

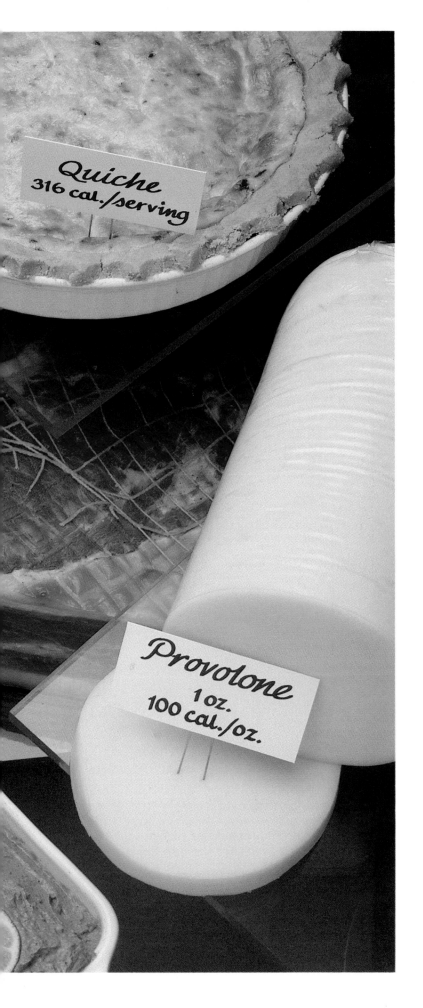

Quiche
316 cal./serving

Provolone
1 oz.
100 cal./oz.

The Calorie Factor

When it comes to your personal fuel tank, some calories will give you better mileage than others.

Imagine what would happen if you filled your car with gasoline every time you used it—but never went very far. Eventually the tank would flood, spilling the excess down the sides. And what if you had to store that extra fuel in gas cans in the trunk, weighing the car down. Now imagine the same thing happening to your body, with food replacing the gasoline. It, too, would be forced to store the overload as excess baggage—human fuel that couldn't be used.

Like your automobile, your body needs a steady but normal supply of fuel to remain in good running order. While your car's fuel is measured in gallons, the body's fuel supply is measured in calories. Unfortunately, too many of us spend our lives "topping off" our personal fuel tanks by consuming too many calories. In fact, there is a single characteristic common to every one of us with a weight problem: We consume more calories than we need.

Yes, calories *do* count. And while counting calories alone cannot permanently solve a weight problem, understanding what a calorie is and how it works is part of the overall weight-control equation. As noted weight-loss expert and nutritionist Jean Mayer, Ph.D., of Harvard University, says, "In the end, you lose weight only by taking in fewer calories than you burn up in activity. No one has yet found a loophole in the laws of nature."

Of course, the trick is to learn how to burn your calories more efficiently. But we've already told you about that in other chapters. Here we're going to tell you how to watch your calories—wisely. Just keep in mind that basing your weight-loss program on calorie charts alone is
(continued on page 126)

Anatomy of a Calorie

A calorie is a calorie is a . . . well, not quite. As we should all know by now, all calories are *not* created equal. They come in three different guises: protein, carbohydrate and the heavyweight of them all—fat. The difference in their appearance is pretty apparent when we stare at them on the plate in front of us. In fact, most of us have our prejudices as to which calories we prefer to have on that plate! But did you ever wonder how these different types of food affect your anatomy *after* they leave the plate and pass the lips?

Well, on first bite, proteins, carbohydrates and fats act pretty much the same. Digestion of all of them begins in the mouth—about 5 percent of all food starches are digested while we chew. But it's when the food hits the stomach that the real digestive process begins. Digestive juices go into full gear, working to break down the food particles. Water, simple sugars and alcohol are absorbed and even more starches are broken down. Proteins are reduced and fats are partially digested. Then it's on to the small intestine, where the proteins, carbohydrates and fats go on their separate ways, as you can see by the illustrations. Yet, when it's all said and done, unneeded proteins, carbohydrates and fats show up as lookalikes—just plain, ordinary padding looking for a comfortable place on the body to take a rest.

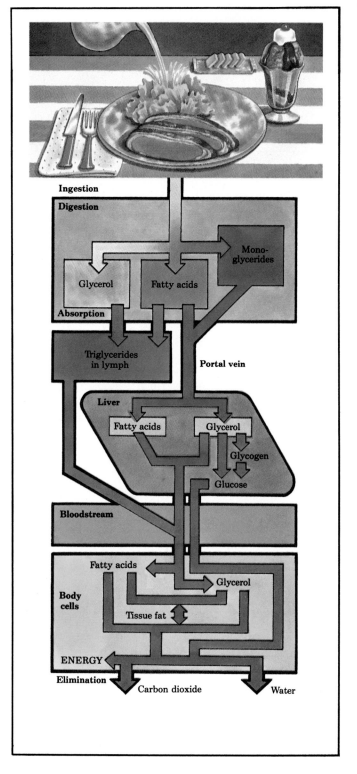

Fats. Fats, in the form of large globules, first enter the small intestine, where bile salts must work to break them down into smaller particles for easier digestion. They then pass through the intestinal wall and eventually enter the bloodstream. While some of these milky-looking fats are used for energy, any excess is stored in body tissues until (if ever) they're called upon for action. (Some fat particles, known as glycerols, are sent directly from the small intestine to the liver, where they are stored for use as energy.)

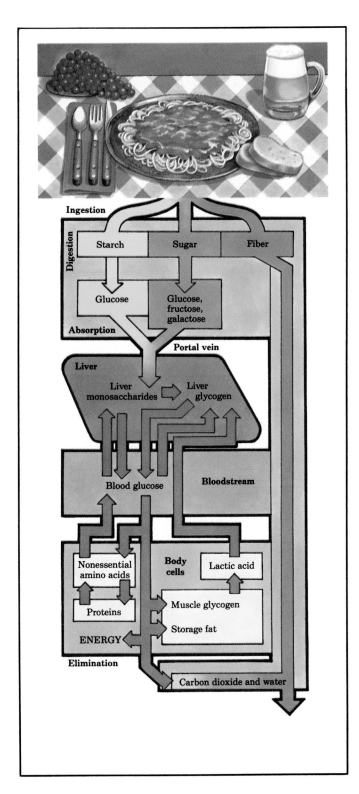

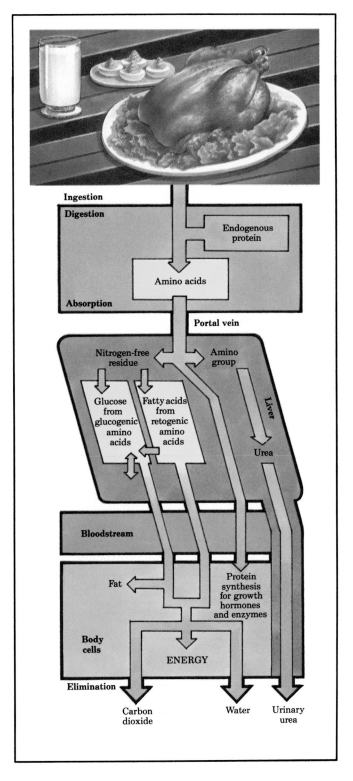

Carbohydrates. When they hit the small intestine, carbohydrates are reduced to absorbable simple sugars. They are then transported through the blood to the liver, where they wait to supply the body with energy. However, if the body can't hold all the carbohydrates in the liver's storage tank, they are converted to fat and sent off to the body tissues for storage.

Proteins. Think of proteins as a large chain of particles called amino acids. When it hits the stomach, digestive juices work on the chain, wearing it down to a smaller chain for passage to the small intestine. Once there, the digestive process works at the chain even more, leaving it nothing more than loose links, which are ready to pass through the body to the circulatory system for immediate use. Any excess is sent to the liver, where it is either stored, sent out to the body for use as energy or—you guessed it—sent to the tissues to mingle with all the other fat.

shortsighted—much like a sailor following the navigational chart and never bothering to look up to see if he's headed for an iceberg.

THE CALORIE CHALLENGE

So, why are we making such a fuss over calories if they aren't the end-all to the weight-loss problem? Because there are about as many misguided notions about calories as there are calories in a hot fudge sundae—literally hundreds. As dietitian and nutrition lecturer Jeanne

Goldberg puts it, "The calorie is the most overworked and least understood word in the dieter's vocabulary." Let's just look at what the Wheat Industry Council discovered when it set out to find what 3,368 people knew about calories. While most of these people said they paid a lot of attention to nutrition labels, it turned out they didn't know a whole lot about calories when it came to guessing the value of certain foods. Asked how many calories are in an 8-ounce glass of whole milk, the participants came up with an average answer of 196 calories. It

Breaking Up a Bad Marriage

Some food "marriages" weren't made in heaven. Here are ideas for foods to substitute or delete to lessen the caloric weight of some well-known couples.

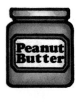 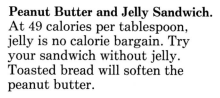

Peanut Butter and Jelly Sandwich. At 49 calories per tablespoon, jelly is no calorie bargain. Try your sandwich without jelly. Toasted bread will soften the peanut butter.

Spaghetti and Meatballs. Each meatball plunks about 78 extra calories onto your spaghetti, not to mention added fat. Pasta with plain tomato sauce will do just fine.

Oil and Vinegar. At 120 calories a tablespoon, oil can weigh down a low-calorie salad. Select tomato juice and herbs or simply lemon juice to accompany the vinegar.

Baked Potato and Sour Cream. Sour cream can "cream" your diet with 52 calories for every 2 tablespoons. Try plain yogurt and save yourself 35 calories.

Popcorn and Butter. With 102 calories per tablespoon, butter can kill this low-cal snack. Instead, sprinkle curry or garlic powder on popcorn.

actually has only 150 calories. Asked how many calories there are in 5 ounces of spaghetti with tomato sauce, they came up with 394 calories, which really tops its true value of only 163 calories. (No wonder spaghetti has a bad reputation for being a fattening food!)

Such poor perception does not surprise a lot of weight-loss specialists. Beverly Keefer, Ph.D., a psychologist and the director of the eating disorder program of the department of medicine at Temple University, Philadelphia, believes that there are other blind spots people have when it comes to calories. Often, she finds, people are anxious to learn the calorie counts of "good" foods like broccoli or white chicken meat but neglect to learn the number of calories in ice cream, candy bars and similar "bad" foods. They also do not pay close enough attention to portion sizes. While the ordinary household does not have precision scales that can measure food portions down to the "nth" calorie, it's not hard to figure out that a slab of beef you buy at the butcher shop is not going to squeeze into the nutritionist's ver-

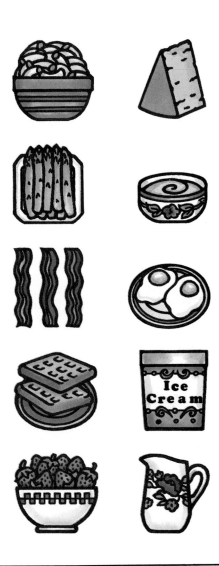

Macaroni and Cheese. The cheese half of this old pair adds about 254 calories to the average serving. How about a cold pasta salad with seafood or vegetables?

Asparagus with Hollandaise Sauce. A half cup of asparagus with a tablespoon of hollandaise is 96 calories. But skip the sauce and you can shear 84 calories off that tally.

Bacon and Eggs. This team can cost your breakfast 275 calories if you eat 3 slices of bacon and 2 eggs. Slice bacon from this popular A.M. pair and save yourself 109 calories.

Waffles and Ice Cream. A helping of waffles and ice cream stacks up to 415 calories. Why not have one without the other? The waffles have 280 calories; the ice cream has 135.

Strawberries and Cream. Some things are just better plain, like fresh strawberries. Three tablespoons of whipped cream add 78 calories, turning this 45-calorie-a-cup treat into a dietary disaster.

sion of a 3-ounce serving. (That's why it is important to pay close attention to the portion sizes specified in a calorie table. When it says 3 ounces, it means precisely that amount.)

Dr. Keefer says she also finds that those wanting to lose weight often have mistaken notions about exactly how fast they will shed pounds if they cut calories. "They have the unrealistic idea that if they eat 800 calories a day, they're going to lose 5 pounds a week," she explains.

Unfortunately, weight loss isn't that easy. In order to be a little more realistic about calories and the role they play in weight loss, let's backtrack a bit for a mini-course on calories.

Calorie-Counting Confusion

So you want to find out how many calories are in a carrot. That's easy enough, you reason. Just look it up in a calorie chart. And what do you find? Well, in one book you'll find a raw carrot contains 30 calories. In another, it has 21. How about cornflakes? One book puts them at 97 calories a cup, but they're listed at 105 calories per 1⅓ cup in another. With the myriad of calorie guides, dictionaries, cookbooks and diet plans on the market today, keeping up with your calories can be downright confusing!

However, you'll be glad to know there is a publication you can depend on for consistency. The U.S. Department of Agriculture (USDA) publishes the "bible" of calorie guides, known as *Agriculture Handbook No. 8*, which is kept up-to-date to reflect changes in eating habits as well as new developments in the way foods are grown. If you would like to obtain a dependable calorie chart based on this handbook, write to the USDA for a booklet called, "Calories and Your Weight." It is available for $3.75 from the Superintendent of Documents, U.S. Government Printing Office, Washington, D.C. 20402 (specify this pamphlet by title and also note that it is number AIB-364).

So, how many calories does a carrot really have? Turn to the chart in chapter 10 to find out.

ALL CALORIES ARE NOT CREATED EQUAL

A calorie, as we explained, is simply a measurement of the amount of heat or fuel food supplies to the body. To be more precise, there are calories and there are kilocalories. Scientists use the calorie—referred to as the "small" calorie—in the laboratory. A kilocalorie is the amount of heat needed to raise the temperature of a kilogram of water—slightly more than a quart—by 1 degree centigrade. Somewhere along the line, the "kilo-" was dropped and we now simply use calorie when discussing energy values of food.

One cup of whole milk, for instance, contains 150 kilocalories, or enough to increase the temperature of 150 quarts of water by 1 degree. A cup of tomato juice contains only 46 kilocalories, or the energy to raise the temperature of 46 quarts of water by 1 degree. Therefore, even though these drinks are seemingly "equal"—a cup each—milk supplies the body with more fuel to burn. Or, to put it another way, the milk supplies more fuel which will be stored as fat if the body is being fed more than it needs.

The method of calculating calories hasn't changed since the mid-1800s, when Edward Frankland, a London scientist, invented the "bomb calorimeter," the device scientists still use to do the calorie measuring we just described. But it was Wilbur Atwater, Ph.D., a scientist with the U.S. Department of Agriculture, who fine-tuned the technique and determined the calorie value of the three basic food components we know today: proteins, fats and carbohydrates. He found that calorie values were higher for animal foods, such as meats, and much lower for fruits and vegetables. By averaging out the fuel values for typical foods, Dr. Atwater figured that each gram of protein and each gram of carbohydrate contain 4 calories. But each gram of fat contains 8.9 calories—more than twice the calories of protein and carbohydrate. Converted another

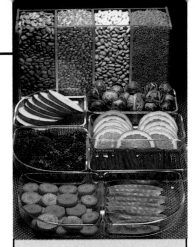

way, each ounce of pure protein and carbohydrate contains 113.6 calories and each ounce of pure fat contains a whopping 252.8 calories! And that's why a glass of milk, which comes from an animal and contains 8.59 grams of fat, has more calories than a glass of tomato juice, which comes from a plant and has 2.2 grams of fat.

These figures, in many ways, are the crux of calorie counting. It all boils down to the fact that some foods are "calorie dense" while others are not. When you eat fats, you're getting more than your fair share of calories per portion. Take a 1-ounce serving of fat-dense walnuts—only 14 walnut halves. They contain 185 calories. You would have to eat almost three slices of whole wheat bread, high in fiber and low in fat, to equal that amount. So while the walnuts are small to the eye, they are big to the body's inner calorie calculator.

That, in a nutshell, is what's wrong and right with our diets. If you aim for a balance of fats, proteins and carbohydrates that minimizes fat-dense foods in your diet, you won't go wrong at the scale. Nutritionists and weight-control experts advise that a proper diet contains 20 to 30 percent fat and 12 percent protein, with the remainder predominately unrefined, fiber-rich, complex carbohydrates. Unfortunately, most people don't follow this advice. The typical American diet is too high in fat—about 40 percent of total calories—and much too low in complex carbohydrates. To keep your body working at peak performance, strive for the food distribution ratio the experts recommend.

GET INTO CALORIE BALANCE

There is another huge piece of the weight-control puzzle you will need to consider—average daily caloric needs. The number of calories your body needs to get through a day depends on many factors—body size and composition, health status, basal metabolic rate (the level of

energy you need to support involuntary body processes such as breathing) and, of course, physical activity. Someone with a larger body size, for instance, needs more fuel to power larger organs and warm up a greater skin surface than a petite person does. Generally speaking, to figure your basal metabolic rate you should allow about 10 calories a day for each pound if you're a woman and 11 calories for each pound if you're a man. That number decreases slightly with increasing age.

When trying to reduce, many folks have a tendency to cut back their calorie intake too severely, under the misguided notion that the more they starve themselves, the faster they'll lose weight. As you've already learned, this is a bad idea. When cutting back calories, nutritionists consider around 1,500 a day (for women) to around 2,000 or more a day (for men) a safe range. Anything below 1,200 is ill-advised. A diet under this amount will almost surely not contain an adequate amount of vitamins and nutrients. In addition, eating too little causes fatigue. And, as you learned in chapter 5, deprivation will only lead to overeating later on.

EAT THE WHOLE DAY THROUGH

The number of calories you consume isn't all that counts, nutritionists say. According to Dr. Isobel Contento, studies show that *how often* you eat may matter just as much. If you consume all your calories at one sitting as opposed to spreading them out over the course of the day, your body, feeling it's in semistarvation, will store more calories as fat, says Dr. Contento. So, if you're hoping to lose weight, don't adopt a starve-and-then-cram-in-one-meal approach. It's bound to work against you.

It appears that how you spread out your caloric intake during the day counts, as well. Studies indicate that those who eat heavy in the morning and light at night have a better chance of losing weight than those who scrimp at breakfast and lunch so they can have a bigger

Fiber Helps Cut Calories

The reason high-fiber foods are good for the dieter goes beyond the fact that they fill you up and take longer to eat. They also have an effect on the way your body digests calories. One study found that fibrous foods in the diet actually reduced the extent to which calories were absorbed from food.

Why does fiber have this calorie-zapping quality? Well, besides providing bulk, it also helps escort dietary fats through the digestive system before they have a chance to be totally absorbed. Whole grain cereals and breads, pasta, beans and vegetables will give you the fiber to battle those calories.

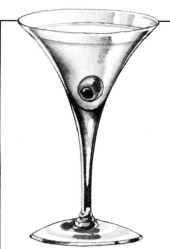

The Truth about Fat and Alcohol

How do alcohol calories differ from food calories? Alcohol calories, you may be surprised to learn, don't turn into fat in your body the way food calories do. Nevertheless, this is nothing to cheer about, for drinking alcohol *can* help make you fat. For one thing, alcohol calories *are* used by the body for energy. And when it comes to a source for fuel, the body always turns to alcohol calories first. So, while your body is burning alcohol for energy, your food calories are left with little or no work to do. The result: *They* turn into fat.

meal later. In one study, volunteers who consumed their calories at breakfast all shed pounds. Yet when they ate the same number of calories at the evening meal, they lost less weight; some even gained. One reason timing counts is that digestion does not peak until some 7 hours after eating. So, if you consume most of your calories during the evening meal, you'll be digesting it while you sleep and your metabolism is at its *slowest*—a prime time for storing fat.

STAYING ON TRACK

Now that you have garnered the basics of calories, where do you go from here? First, recognize that knowing calorie counts for your foods is one thing; doing something constructive about it is yet another. Although paying attention to calories is important, it is still only one component of a good diet plan.

"If you can't say no to Aunt Flossy when you're visiting and she offers you a piece of chocolate cake, it doesn't matter if you know a slice of her chocolate cake is 450 calories," says Dr. Keefer.

You will need to remember several tips as part of a calorie-watching strategy and also be wary of some typical pitfalls.

- Don't lose track of your calories. Many people count breakfast, lunch and dinner rigidly but then fail to include foods eaten late at night or while preparing meals. These can easily add several hundred calories to your total daily intake.
- Take visible fat off your meats. Using a paring knife, take a minute to slice off the fat. The fat not only supplies unnecessary calories, as Dr. Mayer points out, but taking the time to dissect it slows down your eating process.
- Count *all* the calories for ingredients you add in preparing a food, and in garnishes, condiments and similar add-ons. Dr. Mayer offers the example of the baked potato, a

filling 145 calories. Mash it with some cream, and the dish is suddenly 200 calories; start adding butter and the count gets higher and higher. Foods in their simplest form are most often the lowest in calories.

- Remember, condiments do contain calories. One tablespoon of butter, something we often add with little thought to baked fish or a dish of vegetables, has 102 calories. A tablespoon of tartar sauce plunks an additional 74 calories onto fish. A tablespoon of jam or preserves adds 54 calories. So even though minuscule in serving size, such sauces, creams and flavorings are hefty when it comes to affecting the number of calories we consume.

SPEND YOUR CALORIES WISELY

What if someone handed you a big wad of cash so you could go on a shopping spree? Would you blow it quickly on a one-shot-and-done item or would you shop around and spend it wisely on several things so you'd get the most for your money? You can pose the same question to the way you "spend" your calories. You could splurge on a few foods that may tempt you—a couple of colas or a dish of ice cream—but these won't fill you up, physically or nutritionally. But if you really want to make your calorie count stretch far, some foods are just plain better than others for providing the most nutrients and satisfaction for the least calories.

Fish is one of your best investments as an entree, especially if you bake or broil it, plain, without butter. Three ounces of baked flounder is only 67 calories. And most types of fish are low in fat. Tuna, flounder, halibut and perch are your best bets.

Among vegetables, there are several that have high nutrition/low calorie ratios. A cup of broccoli, for instance, contains a whopping 3,880 units of vitamin A and lots of vitamin C and B vitamins, all for a tiny 40 calories. Kale similarly provides huge amounts of A and C, plus calcium, for only 44 calories per cup. Another low-calorie goodie that can keep you munching quite awhile with few calories is a green pepper. It, too, is rich in vitamins A and C, and one large pepper contains only 36 calories.

Tofu is another calorie counter's friend, for it offers an excellent way to get away from red meat. For a small number of calories, it has plenty of protein and is high in iron and calcium. One serving, about 4 ounces, will set your calorie count back by only 86 calories. For that number of calories, you'd only get 1¾ ounces of lean ground beef, so you can see how tofu is a dietary bargain.

THE CALORIE COUNTDOWN

There's an easy way to cut back on calories without ever having to feel hungry, deprived or even like you're on a diet.

The simple truth is that a pound of fat is equal to 3,500 calories. So, in order to lose a pound, you must give up 3,500 calories beyond what you need to maintain your current weight. That sounds like a heavy-duty chore—if you try to tackle it quickly. The idea, however, is to do it gradually. If you cut out just 300 calories a day from your diet—say the piece of pastry you eat at the office each morning—you can lose a pound every 10 days. Cut back 500 calories a day, and you will slim down by about a pound a week, or 10 pounds in just 2½ months. (Increasing your activity through exercise can help use calories, too). If you change the "little-splurge-today, little-less-tomorrow" way of thinking common to calorie counting, and instead take simple steps to steadily cut a small number of calories each day, the results will soon be noticeable.

It can be as easy as this—a husband and wife normally have one sausage link and two pancakes apiece at breakfast. If they decide to share one link and make only three pancakes instead of four—splitting the third pancake—they each have shaved 163 calories.

Little Tricks to Trade Off Calories

The art of cutting calories comes down to making little changes more than attempting wholesale avoidance of foods. Such "pruning" during your daily diet can add up to hundreds of saved calories. Consider that . . .

- drinking coffee *without* a teaspoon of sugar will save you 15 calories per cup and using milk instead of cream will save you 39 calories a cup.
- eating tuna packed in water instead of in oil will cut 159 calories from every 3½-ounce serving.
- mixing tuna fish with a tablespoon of lemon juice instead of mayonnaise will save 96 calories.
- drinking club soda or seltzer water instead of tonic water will save you 70 calories per drink.
- eating ice milk instead of ice cream will save you 85 calories per cup.
- drinking skim milk instead of whole milk will save 64 calories per cup.
- drinking a cup of tomato juice instead of cranberry juice cocktail will save 101 calories a glass.
- using equal parts of oil and vinegar instead of 3 parts oil to 1 part vinegar on your salad will save you 29 calories per tablespoon.
- having a cup of fresh strawberries for dessert instead of a piece of apple pie will save you 359 calories.
- using whipped instead of regular margarine will save you 34 calories per tablespoon.
- eating fruit cocktail packed in water instead of heavy syrup will save you 107 calories a cup.

At lunch, a woman decides to eat two saltines with her daily soup instead of four. She also eliminates her nightly beers on Monday through Thursday evenings—a savings of 600 calories. One less piece of cherry pie can save you 300 calories alone, as can one hot dog on a roll. You'll probably be amazed, once you get started, how easily calories can be pruned. Your body will be the better for it.

9

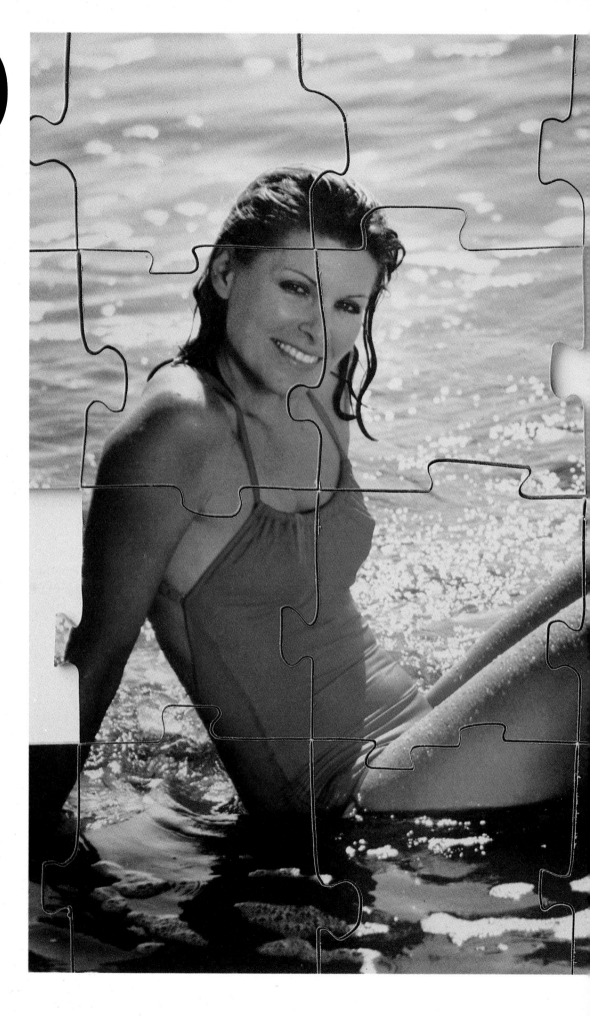

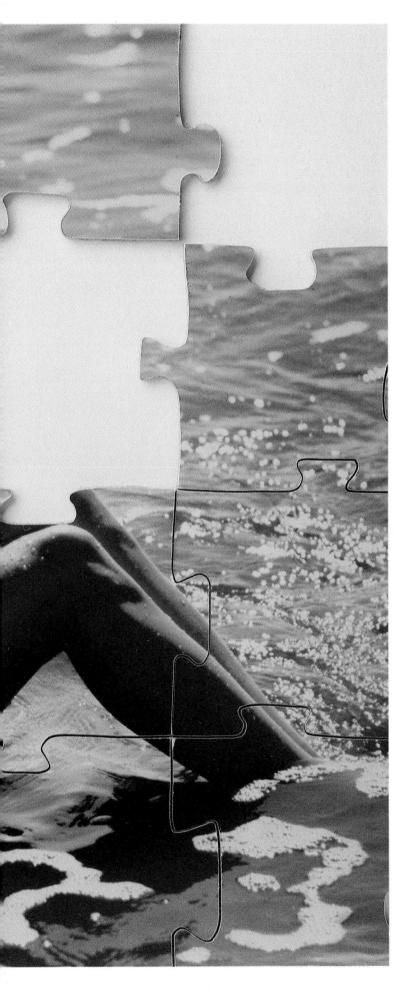

Putting the Plan Together

You have what it takes to lose weight in a healthy, natural and lasting way.

You are on your way to a more beautiful body, a body that will be more fun to live in, a body that matches your spirit and courage, a body that will make every day of the rest of your life more worthwhile.

You have already begun by reading this book, and you may well have already begun to practice some of the suggestions we have made. You have shown that you have the most important quality that you will need to succeed, and that is the willingness to try. If you just keep in mind that willingness is the most important asset you can have, you will know that you can't fail. You can only succeed through whatever steps you make.

Now it's time for you to begin fitting the pieces of this plan into your own lifestyle. The following steps have been gathered here for ease of reference and planning. But don't hesitate to refer back to the sections of this book that deal with these topics more thoroughly. And because there's so much to remember, it's not a bad idea to come back to this list often for reinforcement, too.

Lighten Up to Slim Down. Take it easier on yourself. That's the suggestion of one psychologist who views overweight as often tied to a vicious emotional cycle. The cycle goes like this: An overweight person feels down, eats to feel better, but feels worse instead because the weight problem has only been aggravated. Feeling bad brings on more suffering—and more eating. And this cycle can keep spinning forever unless it is broken.

This isn't to say that overweight is necessarily a sign of emotional trouble. But in this culture which values leanness, it can certainly contribute to a negative self-image.

Some research has shown that there's no difference between fat people and thin people in their ability to cope with life. But it may be that the overweight handle their human problems differently from the lean—namely, by eating. And it's possible that the fat need to be more emotionally sound than the thin if they are to lose. Some recent research has shown that plump psychotherapy patients tend to lose weight even though that wasn't the problem for which they sought treatment. It seems that as their opinion of themselves goes up, their weight goes down.

So here are some simple techniques that may help in your mental battle of the bulge.

Write Yourself Thin. The act of putting pen to paper can help you lose weight. It's not the calories you expend pushing the pen, of course, but the resetting and refocusing of your thinking.

Make a list of the reasons you want to lose weight. This list will no doubt include wanting to look better

The Facts about Fad Diets

Diets that focus on fruit. Diets that promise to keep us slightly stoned. Diets recommended by movie stars. A new fad diet appears every few months, it seems.

But old or new, all fad diets have one thing in common: They promise miracles. They promise that physical and chemical laws will be rewritten in our favor. Flab accumulated over years will vaporize fast in response to the magic wand of enzymes or protein or gallons of water or whatever formula can be foisted upon the gullible.

These diets are related also in the fact that they don't work. To be sure, desperate dieters can lose 10 or even 20 or more pounds, usually by paying a high price in physical and mental well-being. However, much of the lost weight returns shortly after the person leaves the diet, for the loss was mainly water. The rest of the weight comes creeping back almost as quickly because no new eating and exercising patterns were formed and because the body seems to have a kind of built-in defense against such sudden shifts.

The last factor joining fad diets is the risk they tend to pose to health. The hunger pains they cause are minor compared to the dehydration, strain on the heart, kidneys and liver, extreme drops in blood pressure and loss of muscle tissue that are but some of the hazards they pose. Some even kill. Commercial liquid protein diets alone were responsible for 58 deaths in a single year, according to the U.S. Food and Drug Administration.

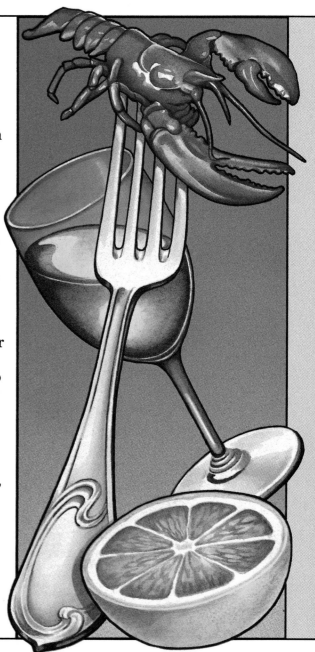

in clothes (and possibly out of them), looking younger, having more energy and feeling better. But make your *own* list. Actually write it out on a piece of paper. Keep it and keep adding to it every time you think of a new reason, no matter how seemingly minor.

This list will help you lose weight by building a kind of mental muscle and reaffirming that you deserve to live the rest of your life in a more attractive, healthy body. It will also help you in those inevitable moments when you can't think of a single reason why it would be better to take a walk down to the park than to eat half of a chocolate cake.

A second list you should make is a list of nonfood rewards, things that you'd like to have, make, buy or do. As you reduce, you should look at this list frequently and choose rewards for yourself. Maybe you'll want to do this on a regular schedule. Maybe you'll give yourself a small reward, such as a notebook to keep track of your exercise progress, each week, and a bigger reward—maybe an additional, nifty

Below you'll find the most popular types of fad diets listed by generic name, and what you can expect from each. Our advice: Keep away from them all.

Type of Diet	What It Is Supposed to Do	What It Really Does	Side Effects
Fruit	Undigested food is thought to cause fat by becoming stuck in the body. Enzymes in fruit are thought to burn fat.	High fruit intake can cause diarrhea. Initial weight loss is due to water loss. Low protein intake can cause muscle loss.	Dehydration, fever, rapid pulse, muscle weakness, mineral imbalances, possibly a fatal drop in blood pressure.
Liquid protein	Said to suppress appetite. Difficulty of digesting protein is claimed to burn more calories.	Causes dehydration. Body burns lean muscle tissue.	Strain on liver and kidneys. Hair loss, constipation, muscle weakness, nausea, neural disorders and gastrointestinal disorders. Death possible.
High protein, high fat, low carbo- hydrate	Deprived of carbohydrates, the body has to burn fat for energy. Aim is to induce ketosis, or high blood levels of ketones. Ketones are formed by incomplete breakdown of fats, and the urinary loss of these unused calories is thought to cause weight loss.	Initial weight loss is due largely to dehydration from water loss. Ketone buildup can cause nausea, which quells the appetite.	Headaches, weakness, nausea, bad breath, frequent urination harmful to the kidneys. High ketone levels are toxic and can lead to death.
High carbo- hydrate, low fat, low protein	Based on the idea that lowering fat in diet will increase oxygen to the body and so reduce disease rates. The diet is very low in protein and fat.	Huge amounts of high-fiber, low-calorie foods are eaten. Since few calories are eaten, weight reduction occurs.	Might be too low in protein for some groups like children or pregnant women. Low fat plus high fiber reduces mineral absorption and may lead to bone softening. Huge amounts of fiber can be dangerous to people with bleeding peptic ulcers or active ulcerative colitis.
Centered on one food	A particular food, like grape- fruit or eggs, or a combination of foods, like bananas and skim milk, is thought to burn fat, increase metabolic rate, remove toxic metabolic products or reduce food intake.	Food choices are so rigidly limited that monotony causes a decrease in food intake. Weight loss is due to reduc- tion of calorie intake.	These diets are nutritionally unbalanced. Depending on the specific diet followed, these side effects may occur: loss of lean muscle tissue, mineral and other nutrient deficiencies.

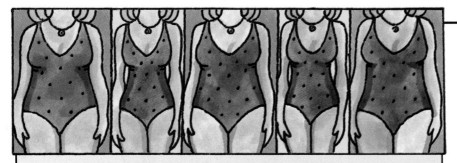

The Ups and Downs
of Yo-Yo Dieting

The Kumquat Diet—nothing but kumquats for 2 weeks. The High Himalayas Diet—you ate on a stepladder. The Ptooey Diet—wish you could forget *that* one.

Each was followed by the inevitable ecstatic end to self-denial. It was goodbye, bean curd—hello, banana cream! And once again you put on the weight you lost.

But you're no worse off, you believe. What you put on this week you can take off again next week. Unfortunately, this quick gain and loss cycle isn't as harmless as you think. It can damage looks, health and psyche.

The horrible fact is that our bodies *build* fat more easily than they *burn* it. Deprived of calories, we convert both muscle and fat to energy. Given excess, our uncooperative metabolism efficiently stores it only as fat. Each time we quickly lose and gain, we look, and are, lumpier and bumpier than ever.

Another health-destroying mechanism operates. During rapid loss, blood pressure plummets alarmingly. During quick gain, it skyrockets, and the heart shows signs of distress—abnormal electrocardiograms, irregular beats, elevated blood cholesterol. Doctors say we may be doing serious, long-term damage to our cardiovascular systems.

Emotionally we suffer, too. Dieting crazily, we are angry, irritable, depressed—notoriously insufferable. Gaining, we are guilty and defensive. Fat once more, we mope around, failures.

But none of this has to happen to you. By following a sensible eating and dieting plan, you can hop off the diet roller coaster forever.

piece of equipment for your hobby—once a month.

Try to make it a practice not to deny yourself anything except too much food. Be good to yourself and generous to yourself whenever possible. Avoid setting up feelings of self-pity because you can't eat like everybody else. Remember, there are a lot of people who also can't eat like "everybody else."

So right now, what would you enjoy? How about a magazine, a hot bath, seeing a movie (skip the popcorn, please), or buying or building a bird feeder? Maybe one of these will strike your fancy or will start you thinking of your own choice. Go ahead and reward yourself right now. You deserve it.

Daydream Yourself Streamlined. Mental images of the self you'd like to be can be a powerful ally in your campaign to change yourself, say weight-loss experts and successful dieters.

Imagine yourself waking up on some sunny morning just before the alarm goes off—in the body that yours could be—and feeling how good it is to be alive. As usual, you're getting up an hour early so that you can take a long, brisk walk. You love listening to the birds as you stride easily along. Your muscles feel strong as you draw in deep breaths of fresh, clean air.

When you get back, you have a hot shower before breakfast and think eagerly about the challenges that you will meet today. You have a feeling of confidence that you will be able to handle whatever comes along.

Forming a mental picture of the person you can be is an important step in the weight-loss process and it is worth your time. You will want to call this picture to mind often to remind yourself of your long-term goal.

"Picture how you want to be and do it," is how one man, who lost almost 150 pounds and has kept it off, puts it. Donald said he used pictures of himself from before the time he gained to help form his image. But if you have always been overweight, you will just have to base your image on your frame. However, make your picture a realistic one, not a vision of Christie Brinkley or Mick Jagger.

And, like Donald, when your friends ask how you're doing, you'll be able to answer honestly, "Great! I can't wait until tomorrow—I'm getting better-looking every day."

You Can't (Help but) Lose with Exercise. In order to solve your weight problem, you must defeat 20th-century technology. Not your fingers but your *feet* must do the walking.

More and more, scientists are recognizing that permanent weight loss is not possible on the basis of calorie restriction alone. At best, dieting alone offers a very temporary solution that is at odds with the body's own powerful mechanism. It's no wonder that at least nine out of ten dieters regain lost weight within months.

But evidence grows daily that *exercise* can influence what scientists call the "setpoint," a metabolic monitor that seeks to hold your weight steady. Exercise, it turns out, is the only "wonder pill" for weight loss.

The trouble is, many of us have learned to hate exercise—the more so as we got fatter. But if we want to lose permanently, we must find a way to turn that around. You are not alone if you hate exercise. The word itself has connotations of smelly sweat, pain, aches and embarrassment for many of us. But it need not—though you may have trouble believing that until you try it the right way. Exercise has almost magically enjoyable properties for those who have overcome their prejudices toward it and found ways of incorporating it into their lives.

You will find that exercise can perform seemingly contradictory wonders—it can calm you, energize you and help you think out the difficulties in your life. It can make you feel better about yourself almost at once. It offers true instant gratification to the child in all of us—and an opportunity to play.

Start slowly on whatever program of exercise you choose, and listen to your body as you do. Don't be self-conscious. Most people who see you, even those who wisecrack, are envious and impressed that you are doing something good for yourself.

Keep a Food Diary. An honest, accurate and complete list of everything you eat—every little

Is Dieting Taboo for You?

Some people should not attempt to lose weight at all. Others should do so only after an in-depth conversation with their doctor. If you are overweight, here's information to help you decide if a program that includes calorie cutting is in your best interest.

Don't diet to lose if you are a nursing mother or if you're pregnant. If you are diabetic, any alteration in your exercise and diet plans should be closely monitored by your physician. Anyone with heart, lung, liver, kidney, pancreas or other organ disease should discuss any proposed dietary changes with a physician before beginning. No one with metabolic or endocrine disorders should diet without getting expert medical advice. And high blood pressure should also signal "Stop—proceed only after consulting a doctor."

nibble—and when, where and why you ate it can be a priceless asset in the work of reshaping your body.

Most people, it seems, have very inaccurate ideas about what they eat—even where they eat. Doctors have found, for instance, that overweight people on a carefully monitored diet of only what they say they eat invariably lose weight.

Many of us tend to underestimate by a good bit the number of calories we take in. We forget the bits of cheese that get chomped while we're making the sandwich. We forget to tally the soft drinks we swallow, though they add hundreds of calories a day. We totally forget that 1,000-calorie visit to the doughnut shop, because we ate the doughnuts in our car.

An accurate, painstaking food diary puts us in touch with our true intake and the conditions under which it takes place. We start to notice when we are eating without hunger. Perhaps we begin to think of what we might do instead. In short, we focus a steady light on our eating habits, and though we thought we knew them well, the results are almost always surprising.

A food diary is such a tremendous learning experience that many people lose simply from keeping one. To pay attention to our eating habits, it seems, is to modify them.

(continued on page 140)

High-Tech Diet Aids

Push a button to lose weight. That may be the appeal behind some weight-loss gizmos. Still, any kind of treat that helps you stay involved with your weight-loss program is a toy that may well be worth your money. (Check retail stores in your area for current availability.)

But don't forget that low-tech—inexpensive or make-it-yourself—rewards also can be reinforcing. A pretty notebook to keep track of your exercise, a neat little 1- to 16-ounce scale for your kitchen countertop, a pair of jeans in a smaller size—these, too, are diet aids.

But whatever fits your budget, do encourage the toy-loving child in you to think of creative ways to help you lose weight. And happy shopping!

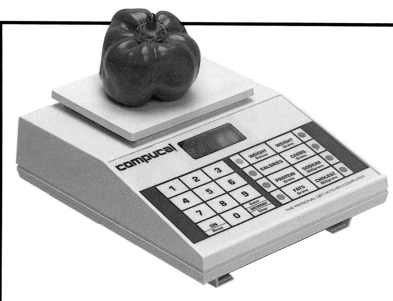

Compucal

The overweight frequently lie to themselves about how much they eat, psychologists say. (A melon-size apple will be called medium-size, for instance.) Compucal can help you get honest. A cross between a scale and a simple computer, it reveals close-to-exact calorie, carbohydrate, fat, sodium, protein and cholesterol counts for foods from abalone to zweiback. The approximate $135 retail price tag (more for batteries and/or AC adapter) would inspire most consumers to use it. It also has a memory unit to keep track of calorie consumption for up to 9 people.

Seca Scale

Unlike that $7.98 scale from the dime store, this all-steel beauty won't subtract 10 pounds when you lean to the left or give 3 different weights at 2-minute intervals. The makers guarantee the Seca to be accurate for 3 years to plus or minus 1 percent of your body weight. But at about $130, you ought to be able to expect it to last a lifetime.

Fitness 3 Micro Computer

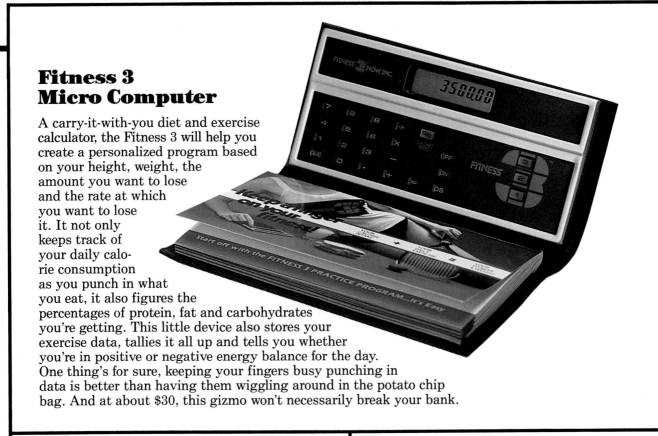

A carry-it-with-you diet and exercise calculator, the Fitness 3 will help you create a personalized program based on your height, weight, the amount you want to lose and the rate at which you want to lose it. It not only keeps track of your daily calorie consumption as you punch in what you eat, it also figures the percentages of protein, fat and carbohydrates you're getting. This little device also stores your exercise data, tallies it all up and tells you whether you're in positive or negative energy balance for the day. One thing's for sure, keeping your fingers busy punching in data is better than having them wiggling around in the potato chip bag. And at about $30, this gizmo won't necessarily break your bank.

Cal Count

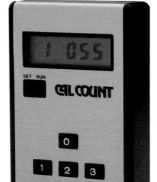

Worn on your body, this ingenious little gadget tells you with near precision how many calories you're burning at any given moment. Its inventor, a professor of biomedical engineering, says Cal Count has been tested against the best laboratory equipment and has proved itself accurate to plus or minus 5 percent. It's definitely an intriguing toy, though you may have to move it around your body to get accurate readings for different exercises. However, you may find facing the awful truth about how few calories you're using each day distressing. The inventor says most folks are surprised. You might want to consider sharing this device with some friends, because getting flabbergasted by your low calorie output costs about $80.

Original Salt Meter

"May I sit near an outlet, please?" That might be your opening line to the headwaiter if you acquire this machine. Plug it in and poke its probe into your chow, liquid or solid, for a meter readout on salt content. Those unfamiliar with how much sodium there is in common foods will be astounded by the results of their tests. Cheddar cheese, for instance, has more than 175 milligrams in a single ounce. Even milk is high in sodium. But you'd need a near-professional interest in salt content to spend roughly $80 when a pocket guide would serve nearly as well.

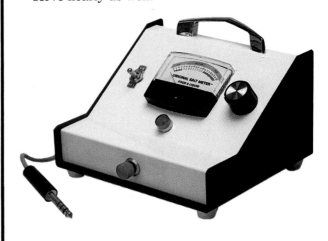

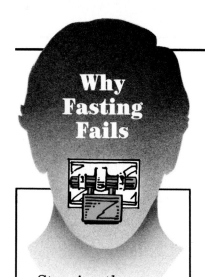

Why Fasting Fails

Starving the over-weight—a method politely called putting them on a fast—is one of many schemes for reducing the obese based on a simple principle: When people don't eat, they lose weight. But there's another principle that fasters shouldn't overlook: When people don't eat, they lose *health*. Fasting can cause metabolic imbalances in levels of heart-nourishing minerals called electrolytes—threatening organ damage and even death. And fasters lose huge amounts of muscle, not just fat.

Some common problems that have been reported are nausea, hair loss, dry skin, muscle cramps, persistent vomiting, softening of bones, halitosis, fatigue and loss of libido.

Face Food Facts. To lose weight, you must take in fewer calories than you burn. It takes approximately 3,500 calories to build a pound of human fat. So, obviously, to lose a pound that number of calories must be eliminated from your diet.

But if this calculation spells H-U-N-G-E-R to you, you're on the wrong track. What you're after in this plan is a *slow* elimination of calories that you really won't miss. Cutting out half a Danish at snack time, ten cashews in the evening and one small bunch of grapes from your daily intake will give you about a 300-calorie deficit—just about the right amount to get rid of daily.

Make calorie charts required reading. Get to know the surprising facts on some of your favorite foods. See if you can't agreeably trade some high-calorie foods for lower-calorie ones without any loss of pleasure. Perhaps you'll discover lower-calorie foods you'll like even better.

Plan for Success. Having a plan can aid your efforts to reshape. If you know what you are going to eat at a certain time, it's less likely that you'll get overhungry—a great danger to those trying to control their intake of calories. It's also less likely that you'll fall into the snack trap.

Not that you shouldn't allow yourself snacks. They can be in your plan, too. If you *plan* on eating a piece of fruit at midmorning, it's less likely that you'll find a giant Hershey bar in your hand then.

Planning can also help make sure you have time to exercise and have made peace with your family, if that's necessary, over that use of your time.

Planning is not meant to suggest rigidity—unless that's what you personally need. Planning merely means making it possible and likely that you will eat and work out in the new way that you want to. And don't forget to put some rewards into your plan!

Be a Supermarket Warrior. Your friendly neighborhood supermarket can be a dieter's enemy. It has been designed to trick, cajole and entice you into buying high-calorie, low-nutrient foods. But you are going to be your own knight in shining armor to defeat the supermarket menace. Here are a few simple rules to help you emerge victorious, bearing healthy foods and not junk.

- Never enter the supermarket hungry.
- Have a list and buy only what is on your list.
- Leave the kids and their demands at home.

If all else fails, don't be shy about asking your mate or a reliable friend to do your shopping. Real friends will spare you the "treats" that add to your fat burden. Remember, it's you against the best minds of Madison Avenue, and you need all the help you can get.

Use the Weigh-Less Savings Plan. Many an urge to eat is triggered not by hunger but by thirst, boredom, loneliness, anger or any feeling of discomfort, major or minor, physical or mental.

Of course, those of us who want to lose weight want to respond to the desire to eat only when the feeling is genuine food hunger. But many of us are not adept at those distinctions. Our almost automatic response to the desire to eat is to do so.

Mark Bricklin, executive editor of *Prevention* magazine and author of *Lose Weight Naturally,* is a victor over a formerly fat body. He discovered that a 7-minute thinking-it-over break gave him the chance to make an honest determination. More often than not, he found himself involved in something else before the 7 minutes were up—the urge to snack hardly even a memory.

Create a Thin World. You can design an environment that will help you lose weight. From the kind of plates you eat on to the place you designate as your dining area, your setting can help you slenderize.

First, you'll want to eat only at the kitchen or dining room table. From your food diary you probably learned that a lot of your eating was

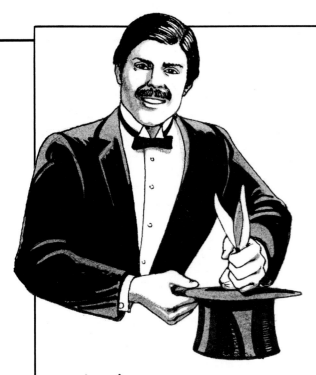

Quick Weight-Loss Schemes

"A rabbit out of an empty hat, folks." That's basically what hucksters offer when they try to sell us quick weight-loss schemes. But even sophisticates occasionally fall for them. The desire to believe in instant, effortless relief from the chronic problem of overweight is so intense that eagerness overcomes doubt and wishfulness defeats reason. We buy the latest magical formula. Our bodies get thinner temporarily, if at all. What gets fatter is the hucksters' wallets. So, if you have been thinking of trying some abracadabra potion, pill or panacea for weight loss, perhaps the list below will save you money, time and trouble.

Spirulina

A form of blue-green algae, this nasty-smelling and nasty-tasting stuff was dieters' pet panacea for a while. Though it's harmless in small quantities, say doctors, it's also worthless as an appetite soother and a ridiculously expensive form of protein at about $4 an ounce.

Glucomannan

Advertised as a "weight-loss secret of the Orient," glucomannan probably should have stayed there. Its sellers claim it fills you up and helps food pass through you quickly. They're the only ones who believe it—if they do. Doctors don't.

L-ornithine and L-arginine

Extremely expensive, these amino acids, when taken together, have been touted with the claim that they stimulate the production of growth hormones in adults, and this causes weight loss. Hogwash, say reputable health professionals.

HCG: Human Chorionic Gonadotropin

A hormone extracted from the urine of pregnant women, shots of HCG have been ballyhooed as an aid to melting the pounds away. Though it may helpful in treating infertility, it's worthless for weight loss, according to the American Medical Association.

Diuretics

People who truly need diuretics are rare indeed, say reputable physicians. To use them for temporary weight loss is a dangerous abuse of these drugs, especially for people on low-calorie diets, doctors say.

Diet Pills

Physicians now recognize that weight loss achieved on drugs can only be maintained on drugs, sometimes on ever-increasing doses of these often-addictive substances. Most doctors now regard them as inappropriate and unsafe for weight loss, and at least one state has made prescribing them for that purpose illegal.

If you want to lose body fat, say physiologists, it's important that you continue reducing calories over a long stretch of time. Tests of dieters have shown that the percentage of fat lost goes up after a period of dieting. In the first few days of dieting, virtually all you lose is water.

It's important, too, that you combine your calorie cutting with exercise, which protects against loss of lean muscle tissue. In one experiment, illustrated in the chart below, the composition and amount of weight lost during a 24-day period on a 1,000-calorie diet with an enforced exercise period of 2½ hours per day was recorded. Note that marked fat loss does not take place until the diet has been under way for 11 days.

happening in odd places—in the car, in front of the TV, in the kitchen, even in the bathtub. These were locations where food seemed to sneak into your mouth. You were so oblivious to it that the food diary was absolutely a revelation.

Well, now you're going to deal with that by decreeing those areas off-limits. You want to eliminate those unconscious eating moments, so you're going to eat only when sitting at the table, and slowly, savoring each bite. One of your aims is to become super-conscious of your eating.

You'll also want to make the table setting give you cues to slow down. Formally arranged food served on elegant dinnerware with a wide border is likely to encourage the kind of behavior you want to develop. Rough stoneware and pewter suggest hearty feasting, a no-no for the weight conscious.

Try to put all the food you're going to eat on your plate at the start. Family-style service, with platters and bowls of food on the table, only encourages those second and third helpings that we take almost without noticing. And around

the house, get rid of those decorative nut bowls and candy dishes.

All cues to stock fattening foods—like empty cookie jars and cake savers—should be put far out of sight in the back of a bottom cabinet. Or if your family demands a full cookie jar, place it out of sight and in a hard-to-reach spot.

But ask yourself if those cookies really are for the kids. Martha's excuse for keeping a huge bin of Oreos around was that the kids demanded them, and she felt they deserved a treat occasionally. But when she really looked at her own behavior with the help of her food diary, she saw that the kids were getting cookies occasionally while she was eating them *steadily* every morning after cleaning. Now she buys cookies only from the vending machine, in individual-serving size. She puts each child's name on the packs as soon as they're in the house.

Martha has also started keeping jars of washed carrot sticks in the refrigerator so they're the first thing she sees when she just "happens" to open the door. Her food scale is in an obvious place on the counter. And on the outside of the refrigerator, she has a picture of a slim female jogger silhouetted against a sunset.

Slow Down to Shed Pounds.
Behavioral scientists have discovered that fast eating is one of the characteristics that tends to set the overweight apart from the thin. (When you were keeping your food diary, you might have noted this characteristic about yourself.)

Fortunately, this is something you can change, and it can make a big difference in your weight. You have already made the first step, which is awareness of the habit.

Now practice doing it differently. After each bite you take, put your fork down on your plate and chew your food thoroughly. Although it will seem unnatural at first, you will find that you enjoy the smaller amount you are eating more and that you seem to fill up on less.

There's another time trick to keep in mind. Physicians have determined that it takes about 20

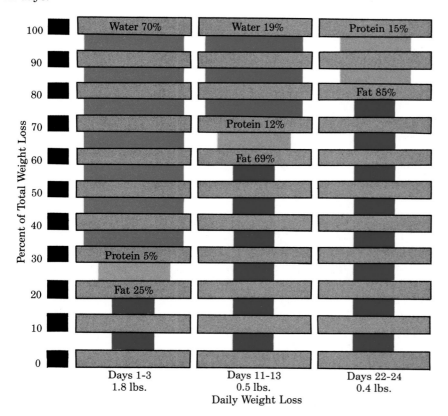

Water 70% | Water 19% | Protein 15%
Protein 12% | Fat 85%
Fat 69%
Protein 5%
Fat 25%

Percent of Total Weight Loss

Days 1-3
1.8 lbs.

Days 11-13
0.5 lbs.

Days 22-24
0.4 lbs.

Daily Weight Loss

minutes after we eat for a feeling of fullness and satisfaction to arrive. So you can help yourself lose by leaving the table when you are finished with one plateful. Do something else for a while, and the urge to eat more, particularly dessert, will pass.

Be Your Body's Buddy. This strategy to lose weight is more than a war on fat. It is a war on the factors that made you fat and the start of a road to a new, more vital and healthy way of life. It is not a plan just for today, but for your tomorrows as well. The food and exercise strategy that will help you slim down should also benefit every other facet of your health.

An important part of this plan is how you divide your diet among the food groups. Doctors now suggest that many of us eat far too much fat and also too much protein. Starting now, aim your eating habits so that no more than 30 percent of your calories comes from fats, 12 percent from protein and all the rest from the complex carbohydrate group—whole grains, fruits and vegetables, the less processed the better. By emphasizing the complex carbohydrates, you'll automatically cut down on fat and protein.

Conquer Calories with Complex Carbohydrates. This food group has had a dirty reputation with the overweight for years. Baked potatoes were frowned at and spaghetti drew sneers.

But now complex carbohydrates are being introduced into weight-loss schemes. In fact, they have become positively welcome as scientists increasingly report their helpfulness in moderate programs of weight loss. It turns out that the butter and rich sauces that get ladled onto the complex carbohydrates are the real villains in the calorie department.

Complex carbohydrates, particularly the unrefined kind, offer us filling, stomach-satisfying bulk as well as nutritive value.

Let Fiber Fight Fat. Fiber foods offer multiple benefits to calorie counters. Because they are usually unrefined, they can fill you up and still be reasonably low in calories. Generally speaking, they also offer quality for the calories you spend on them—high food value in vitamins and minerals. Vegetables, fruits and whole grains all abound in fiber.

Another benefit of fiber is the ease with which it travels through your digestive tract. A particular type of fiber—bran—is particularly useful at this bulking function. That is, it picks up moisture as it moves along and helps to keep everything else moving along at a nice pace. And a high-fiber diet cuts calorie absorption because it cuts down the absorption of fat. So enjoy a few extra calories' worth of this healthy food without paying the price in poundage.

By the way, if you're wondering about the difference between fiber foods and complex carbohydrates, the answer is that many foods are both. Vegetables, fruit and whole grains fall into both categories, and they are your overall best calorie buy. But don't confuse complex carbohydrates with simple carbohydrates like sugar and honey, which should be on your almost-never list.

Don't Let "Glue Foods" Stick on You. "Glue foods" is the name one weight-loss expert has given to empty-calorie foods, usually the kind that contain a lot of sugar and white flour. Cake, ice cream, pie, cookies, doughnuts—all offer little except calories you don't need or want.

When you are tempted to eat these glue foods, imagine them stuck in ungainly lumps on the parts of your body where you usually gain. When suddenly confronted with a food too rich for your eating program, picture it in some unattractive way. A box of popcorn soaked in butter becomes a box of ants, or a plate of pasta in cream sauce is a mass of worms.

And don't forget about fats and oils, with more than twice the calories of an equal amount of sugar. Your alertness can keep them from pasting themselves on your stomach or hips. Not that you will forswear these foods utterly. But you do want to be in complete, conscious control of when and where you eat them and how much of them you eat.

Beware of False Food Friends. No one had to tell you that potato chips, chocolate cake, and sugary drinks are fattening. But what about a little innocent, unsweetened, fiber-rich dried fruit from the health food store?

Eat four dried peach halves and you've taken in over 100 calories' worth of energy. Nuts, nutritious foods rich in vitamins and minerals, are also rich in oil and thus in calories. Ten cashews—and who can eat just ten?—pack a notable 88 calories.

And what weight watcher hasn't eaten a chef's salad with many feelings of virtue? That virtuous salad, however, may make mincemeat of any diet. It may contain as much as 2,000 calories, more than a whole day's supply for some people who are trying to lose.

So be alert. Don't get tricked by myths. And watch out for the label "diet food." The platter bearing a greasy burger with no roll, creamed cottage cheese and coleslaw may have more calories than a plate of spaghetti. But you can defeat these false food friends by using a reliable calorie guide and by weighing your food until you develop the ability to make an accurate "eyeball" judgment.

Slash Your Salt. You've no doubt heard by now that too much salt contributes to high blood pressure, a factor in heart disease. Overweight or not, many people are discovering that they can live better with a lot less of it—in fact, they may be able to live longer simply by slashing the amount they take in.

Used primarily as a flavoring that has been processed into many foods, an enormous amount of salt has crept into the modern diet. And though our bodies need a small quantity of it to go about their metabolic business, that amount is readily supplied in foods just as they are in their natural state. We need never go near the salt shaker.

Weight watchers have an addi-tional motive for banning that shaker of little white crystals. The more salt we dump into ourselves, the more water we retain. The more water, the more weight. So slowing down drastically on the salt is a simple, safe and healthy way to lose a fast few pounds.

You may even find that with your improved diet, you like the taste of food much better without all that unnecessary sodium.

Ban the Binge. How can binges, those sprees of berserk eating, be avoided?

First, you'll want to avoid extreme hunger. If you associate hunger with losing weight, you've made a bad mental connection, and you need to change that thinking.

Getting overhungry is not virtuous. It is setting yourself up for uncontrolled eating. In fact, sometimes you should eat when you *don't* feel hungry. Scientists tell us that those of us who are overweight may have trouble perceiving or correctly interpreting internal feed-ing cues. That means we may miss a body hunger sign or we may not realize we feel hungry at all—though our bodies are ready for food. This makes it especially important that we follow our eating plans.

The desire to get slimmer faster is destined to make us lose not weight but any resistance to temptation. It is not the way to establish good habits, and it's self-defeating.

Another key to binge control is simply to identify those foods—and almost everyone has them—that set us off on a binge. Whether it's the infamous peanut that you can't eat just one of, or pretzels, or just-baked bread, try to stay away from your trigger foods. Or if the urge is overwhelming, allow yourself to eat only one and then hide the rest. Put them out of sight and out of reach.

Put Time on Your Side. Because everybody hates dieting, it is easy to understand the appeal of lose-it-quick schemes. Even though it may have taken years to build to our present level of overweight, once we decide to do something about it, we

Weight Loss: Going to Extremes

The more bizarre the better, seems to be the standard by which some research physicians judge the methods they concoct to reduce extremely overweight people who fail to lose by natural methods. Justifying the radical and untested nature of some of their procedures, the researchers claim, are the acknowledged health risks faced by "massively" obese people—those who weigh more than double what they should. Nevertheless, such drastic methods of weight loss, particularly surgical ones, do carry their own risks, and an overweight person should think long and hard before becoming a guinea pig for such a "cure."

Stomach Stapling. A surgeon closes off all but a small portion of the stomach with rows of stainless-steel staples. The small intestine is reconnected to this sac. The purpose is to make it impossible for the patient to eat more than a small amount at any one time. Tearing out of the staples is a frequent complication. Vomiting is reported by a large number of patients.

Stomach Balloon. This is just what the name implies. A long tube is inserted through the mouth, then a balloon is placed in the stomach and inflated to prevent the patient from filling the stomach with food. Unable to eat much, the patient loses weight. Some experimenters have reported frequent problems with bursting balloons. Others have encountered difficulties with patients experiencing upper abdominal fullness and pains that mimic heart attack symptoms. Whether or not weight losses can be maintained by patients who have had their eating mechanically obstructed has not yet been determined.

Jaw Wiring. Under local anesthesia, physicians wire the patient's mouth shut so that only liquids can be consumed. Weight loss results. But most studies show an inevitable regain after the wires are removed. Jaw wiring itself has other drawbacks. Severe stiffness of the jaw may result, though it's usually temporary. And the procedure makes no provision for the patient to clear air passages in the event of vomiting.

Suction Lipectomy. In this operation, fat is literally sucked out vacuum-cleaner-style through a foot-long tube inserted through a slit in the patient's skin. The supposed advantage of this method over earlier slice-away-the-flab measures is its lack of scarring. However, cosmetic results are not always good. The area where suction surgery has been performed sometimes looks like a "fallen souffle," according to one observer. Long-term numbness has also been reported.

Intestinal Bypass. This is a surgical procedure in which a length of the small intestine is closed off and the remainder reconnected to form a shorter pathway. Intended to make calorie absorption difficult, this operation also blocks absorption of other vital nutrients like vitamins and minerals. Common side effects that have been reported are weakness, diarrhea and dangerous disturbances in body chemistry. Some observers estimate that serious medical complications have occurred in virtually 100 percent of people subjected to this operation.

want it taken care of yesterday.

But our bodies fight off violent assaults on our weight. Severe calorie restriction has proved to be actually dangerous. And even if you go ahead and risk your life to lose weight, the weight-loss plans based solely on austere calorie consumption are doomed to failure. Because of the slowing metabolic rate and the lack of a real change in lifestyle, such efforts are doomed from the start. They only cause needless suffering. Instead of a quick weight loss, you should set as your goal a *genuine* weight loss that will improve rather than damage your health. And that is a *slow* weight loss. "The longer it takes, the longer it lasts," is one dieter's way of putting it.

Nutrition experts say that by no means should your loss of body fat exceed 2 pounds a week. But successful losers who have managed to stay slim suggest a much less drastic rate—a maximum of 1 pound a week. An even better figure might be 3 pounds a month or about ½ pound a week. If that sounds too slow to you, remember that you are saying goodbye to that fat forever. You are starting a new life.

Maintaining Your Loss

Congratulations! You've reached your goal, the weight you wanted to be. You've uncovered a new you—a you who has the energy to do all the things you want to do and the sense of adventure to try totally new things. A you who can do more than you ever believed possible.

Find Your Daily Number

To keep your weight steady, you must take in the same number of calories that you burn. But just exactly how do you determine what that number is? Choose the lifestyle below that's closest to yours, plug your weight into the simple formula and multiply by the number given. The answer is your daily calorie need.

Extremely Inactive

You have a job that keeps you at a desk virtually all day. You never exercise. Your motto is, "Why walk when I can ride?" You like sports—on TV.090

$$\_\_ \times 13 = \_\_$$

Less Active Than Average

You are sedentary on your job. Less than once a week you bestir yourself for a small amount of exercise. You don't like walking. The elevator is your good friend.

$$\_\_ \times 14 = \_\_$$

Reasonably Active

You take part in an active sport once or twice a week. You also walk. Or your job requires you to exert yourself for at least 15 minutes each day.

$$\_\_ \times 15 = \_\_$$

Very Active

At least 3 times a week, you perform vigorous exercise like running, swimming or handball for an hour. You walk and use stairs. Or hard physical labor fills 40 percent of your workday.

$$\_\_ \times 17 = \_\_$$

Extremely Active

You may be an athlete in training. You run 10 miles a day or perform an equivalent activity. Or your job demands heavy physical exertion from you 70 percent of the time.

$$\_\_ \times 21 = \_\_$$

Yes, that's you reflected in the store window in that sleek new outfit. It's you who is drawing the admiring glances from across the street. It's you who other people now turn to readily for help and advice.

You have learned to think better of yourself, too. When someone tells you how nice you look or remarks on how much weight you've lost, you say, "thank you," and you mean it. You don't say, as you once might have, "Oh, I should have lost it years ago," or "Remember how fat I was?" Or "it was all this diet . . ."

You did it, you unmasked this wonderful new you. And you deserve to praise yourself and be praised by others. You always did.

One of the ways you treat yourself well today—and one of your major finds in your new way of life—is your exercise program. Exercise—remember the horrible associations of pain and boredom that word used to have for you? You can laugh at that view today.

Now you have experienced for yourself the wonderful paradox of exercise—its ability to both soothe and energize you. Its ability to convert negatives—tiredness, crankiness and especially anger—into positives.

Exercise not only helped you become slim, it gave you more vigor, vitality and motivation. You feel younger than you have in years. Appetite suppressant, mood elevator —you would no more think of stopping your aerobic routine than you would trade your new body for your old one.

Eating healthfully has also become something you enjoy. You do it not out of martyrdom but out of self-love. You like the way you feel and look better after a meal of broiled chicken, baked potato with yogurt and steamed broccoli than after a greasy steak, french fries and peas in cream sauce.

You found that you feel just as full and more satisfied after eating right. Now you know that you never have to be hungry on a healthy diet.

Because you have learned your new life habits in a slow and natural way—not dropped a sudden, unnatural 20 pounds on the Doctor's Hollywood Marshmallow Diet—you are well on your way to a lifetime peace pact with your weight. You can declare the Battle of the Bulge over.

CHANGES TO LAST A LIFETIME

The price of freedom from fat, just like the price of liberty, is constant vigilance. Your new habits are just that—new. You may have been living a more healthy life for some months now. But your 12-Twinkies-for-dinner, never-walk-when-you-can-ride lifestyle has roots that may go back decades. So you will want to do some thinking about this phase of weight maintenance that you have entered as a result of your success with weight loss.

First, accept the fact that you are entering another learning period. You know how to lose weight. And your body knows how to be overweight. But you do not yet have much experience living in a well-proportioned, fit body.

If that kind of living sounds like a pleasure, it should. But it isn't a snap. If you think it is, you are setting yourself up to regain.

The statistics on keeping weight off are gruesome. In past studies, it has been discovered that at least 4 out of 5 people who lose put it all right back on. But most of these people lost through pure calorie restriction during times when energy metabolism was understood much less well.

Now new scientific evidence is growing to confirm the principles emphasized in this book—that the only effective way to reduce is a slow program that relies largely on exercise and on a sane, sensible program of calorie intake.

How very difficult it is to maintain a weight loss is shown by the poundage added even by certain experts and authors of diet books. Franklin Cordell, Ph.D., a coauthor of *Psychological War on Fat*, and a veteran of a 60-pound loss and the victim of a 20-pound regain, says maintenance of a loss is difficult because we refuse to acknowledge the difficulty. Thus, we fail to pay attention and our weight starts to creep back up.

"It's almost easier for people to keep losing than it is for them to stabilize their loss," says another psychologist. He suggests that to maintain your weight loss, it is critical to recognize the perilous nature of the task you're facing and keep your weight as a priority in your life—for the rest of your life.

You must resist the natural tendency to let up and relax after having reached your goal. That tendency will lead you slowly but surely down the wrong road. Your old habits come creeping back, and so will the extra inches.

Scientists say that your body itself is trying to sabotage your reduction. Very powerful mechanisms exist to return your weight to its old level. Your body will even turn food into fat more efficiently after you've lost, doctors say.

"It's a magnificent mechanism if you're impressed with the body's ability to regulate itself," says Richard Keesey, Ph.D., who has studied weight loss for many years at the University of Wisconsin. "But it's not such happy news for dieters," he adds.

So know the task ahead of you—and be aware that you will need to keep your figure a top priority if you want to stay slim.

Paying attention to this maintenance phase is just as important as your losing phase, particularly for the first few months. You are going to need to give yourself almost as much care and attention as you did during your loss.

If you have followed the slow, natural, physically active path to losing, you may already be near the balance between eating and exercis-

When Being Thin Isn't 'In'

"You can't be too rich or too thin," goes the wisecrack. Wrong, now say scientists. Too much money might not be hazardous to your health, but being too thin *is*.

That's the conclusion of several researchers, one of whom analyzed more than 16 major, long-term population studies. Premature death, long linked to overweight, was also statistically tied to underweight.

A certain amount of body fat, say researchers and doctors, is essential for the body to function properly—a reason why anorexia nervosa is such a deadly disease.

Doctors warn too that overlean athletic women risk temporary fertility loss. And anyone who loses a lot of weight involuntarily should know it's a red-flag alert that means call your doctor.

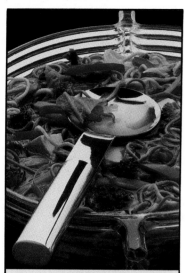

Slurp Yourself Slim

Soup can help you slenderize, researchers have found. It seems people naturally eat hot soup slowly, and eating slowly aids weight loss. Plus, soup provides filling, warming bulk that helps us feel satisfied longer with less.

In a 10-week University of Pennsylvania study, the soup-with-lunch bunch lost 5 percent more of their extra weight than their nonsouping counterparts. But keep calories in mind. Don't let rich cream soups or fatty stocks cut into your losses.

ing that will keep you at the best weight for you. Try keeping your patterns just as they are for another week or two to see if your weight stays steady. If you lose another pound or two, you can begin to think about *gradually* increasing your food intake.

The key word in that last sentence is *gradually*. It is a very human tendency to underestimate what we eat. Scientists restoring dieters to maintenance eating by increments of thirds found that almost none of their subjects needed the last third. They were already taking it in, having overestimated the first two "thirds."

You also don't want to let your level of exercise drop. You'll want to keep getting off the bus one stop early, making your whole wheat bread from scratch and swimming at the Y for ½ hour 3 or 4 times a week—or whatever program you've come to enjoy.

Another key to maintenance in both the eating and exercise departments is to continue planning. Use your food and exercise diaries. The food diary will not only help you gain factual information about the right kind and amount of food for you, it will reinforce positive behavior. Keeping one is psychologically rewarding in itself.

And the same goes for the exercise diary. For example, certain very slow, far-from-professional joggers like to keep track of every split second their bodies are out there moving. It gives them a feeling of satisfaction. And isn't that really what all of this is about?

KEEP REWARDING YOURSELF

It's likely that your rewards have dropped off as your weight has neared or reached your goal. The storm of compliments has trailed off to a flurry. You've purchased most of the new clothes you think you need, so that source of reinforcement has lessened, too.

Now's a good time to remind yourself that keeping your weight at the new level is just as much of an

achievement as losing was. And it very definitely *is* an achievement. It is, in fact, the big test of a successful program of weight loss. And you deserve to keep giving yourself rewards for it.

Keeping track of your weight should be rewarding, too—and if it isn't, then you know it's time to think about stepping up the exercise and looking for a few calories to cut that you won't miss. It's probably a good idea to make a weekly weigh-in a ritual. A midweek morning would likely be the best time to get an accurate fix on how your weight is faring. But bear in mind that poundage is only one way of judging your condition and muscle is heavier than fat. Once more, your mirror is your best friend. The mirror is honest. It's the best check on your new, improved image.

Don't be like Linda, who, though she felt as if she'd traded in her battered bus of a body for a brand new MG, could see only the lumps of ripply fat that stubbornly remained on her hips, not the sleek new lines of the rest of her.

When you look at yourself in the mirror, try to see yourself as others see you. See the fine bulge of a well-toned muscle, the smooth curve where once there was a blob, the beauty of a trim line. Don't focus all your attention on your minor faults. Everyone has them.

If you are really distressed about little pads of fat here or there, you can always increase your exercise. Exercise gives us all another way to get better as we get older. Many of us who were not sports-minded in our teens and twenties—this applies particularly to women—can achieve a level of fitness later in life beyond anything we'd imagined.

Perhaps you were like Stan, who trimmed 150 pounds off a 6-foot frame and has kept his weight at 175 for more than 2 years.

"I couldn't breathe," remembers Stan with a grim laugh. "I sweated a lot. It was terrible. I had nine double chins. I think I carried it rather well, though," he jokes.

Stan has kept his weight down

with a program of rigorous jogging which he enjoys almost on a daily basis. "It keeps me sane," he says. He also eats a sensible diet which does include an allowance of sweet treats like the Pennsylvania Dutch sticky buns he enjoys and earns with his vigorous exercise.

But Stan also rewards himself in other ways, and you should, too. The formerly fat need to remember that they deserve rewards when they are maintaining their new weight just as much as they did when they were losing. Keep your reward list up to date.

Of course, eating right and exercising and having a trim body are their own rewards. But overcoming the temptations of the instant gratification of too many overly sweet or greasy foods requires some fortitude and foresight. You deserve to be rewarded for doing it. Remember always to praise yourself when you do well and not to condemn yourself for slips.

Don't forget to show off your new body. You deserve to be proud of it. Keep adding to your wardrobe. It's one of the most reinforcing things you can do, according to those who have maintained their loss successfully. You're a grownup now, and you don't have to wear your clothes to tattered rags or outgrow them before you replace them. In fact, outgrowing them is precisely what you want to avoid!

Do get rid of your old "fat" clothes, say the experts and winning losers. To keep them around is an implicit admission that you expect to gain the weight back.

Another important thing to remember. Don't expect *too* much from yourself and from life just because you have lost weight. *You* know how much better your life is, how much more you enjoy the simple pleasures today. But losing weight didn't change your life totally. You'll set yourself up to be disappointed if you expect a complete metamorphosis.

Most of all, enjoy yourself and your new body. You've earned every second of the fun!

The 3 P's of Party Preparedness

Some of the people in the photo below will survive the party with their self-respect and calorie counts intact. Others are setting themselves up for failure.

If you think the ones following rigid, self-denying rules—like having only club soda or eating nothing at all—are those who will succeed, you're mistaken, behavioral experts say.

If you want to be a party winner, we suggest you practice the 3 P's of Party Preparedness. First, *prepare* yourself by eating a calorie-conscious meal before you go to the party. If possible and appropriate, bring something with you like a beautiful salad that you and others can enjoy.

Second, *plan* your party responses. Picture the temptations you will face—a laden buffet table, for instance. See the way you want to react, like putting small portions on a small plate. Plan what you'll drink, too. What you should *not* do is plan on denying yourself all treats. Third, *put it off.* Being tempted is not the same as succumbing. Wait a few minutes before you fill up on chocolate mousse, and you may find a little will do. Procrastination can be a winning ploy.

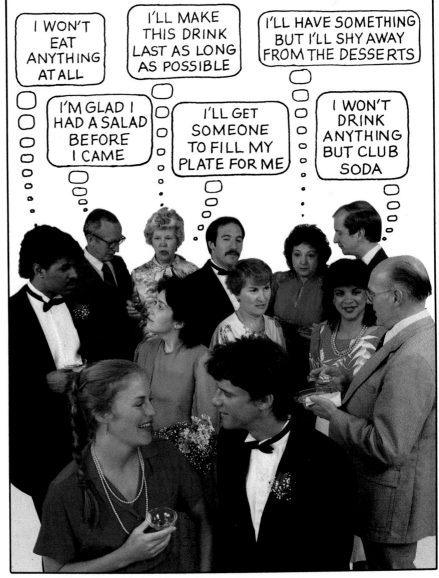

Dieter's Q and A

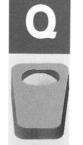

Why is it that it takes me 2 months to lose 10 pounds, but after just one big evening out, the scale says I gained 5 of them back overnight?

Much of this gain reflects additional water. It's not a gain of fat. Unfortunately, not all the 10 pounds you lost was pure fat either, but was also partly water.

Salt intake, hormone levels and exercise all influence the amount of water your body—which is roughly 60 percent water to start with—retains. And many women find they have a monthly gain and loss tied to their menstrual cycle.

But if you have been faithful to a program of reducing calories below your energy needs, your one-night lapse should not prove to be a permanent disaster. Extra exercise can help you shed your water gain more rapidly.

Your frustrating experience points up why the scale is not necessarily the best friend of people who are trying to lose weight. Many who have been doing well give up in despair because of such seemingly irrational and unfair upswings in weight.

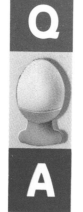

I read in many places that breakfast is very important. But I'm not at all hungry when I get up. How important is it really in terms of my diet and overall health?

If you're one of those people for whom breakfast can spoil an otherwise good day, there's no need to be rigid about a morning meal. That vision of a hearty meal at 7 A.M. suited an era when people already had been laboring in the fields or barn for 2 hours by that time.

Many people do not feel hungry upon first arising. In fact, some people say they can't even give food a thought until they've been up and about for a few hours. If you're such a person, there's nothing wrong with putting breakfast off until midmorning. But don't use it as an excuse to skip breakfast altogether. As you let yourself get too hungry, your blood sugar level will fall and you may find yourself feeling tired and irritable and perhaps craving a sweet for that quick pick-me-up. That's why so many people fall into the midmorning coffee-and-doughnut snack trap. Instead, greet those first pangs with something healthy—a piece of fruit, whole wheat toast or a small piece of cheese.

There is something you *should* know about breakfast. Some researchers have found that while eating a big meal at night tends to add pounds, that same calorie-laden meal in the morning doesn't make for a weight gain. One reason is that digestion doesn't peak until about 7 hours after the last swallow. If most calories are eaten at the evening meal, digestion then occurs when you're sleeping, the time when your metabolism is at its lowest. So, that old adage that tells us to breakfast like a king, lunch like a prince and dine like a pauper seems to be finding solid backup in modern nutritional discoveries.

Everyone seems to have a different opinion about how often I should weigh myself— every day or once a week. When *should* I get on the scale?

Maybe never. This idea may seem radical at first, but it's really common sense. After all, when you see a good-looking man, you don't say to yourself, "Wow, what a body! About 180, I'd say." Nor does a beautiful woman inspire the thought, "I'll bet she tips the scale at a nifty 125." Obesity can't be measured by a scale. It's how you *look* that counts the most. So, it only makes sense to let your mirror be your measure.

"If you have a pair of jeans that are really tight, you can use them as a fat-loss indicator," says Dennis Remington, M.D., director of the Eating Disorder Clinic at the Brigham Young University Student Health Center. "Try them on and evaluate how they fit. Put them away and don't wash them or wear them. Try them on every few weeks and compare the fit to the previous trial. This may show a real change in your body when you might otherwise be discouraged by the scales."

Of course, the no-scale method demands rigorous honesty. You have to be able to admit why you've been avoiding those blue jeans. You have to be willing to look at your reflection objectively rather than wishfully. One trick you might try: Cut eyeholes in a paper bag. Put it over your head before you examine your full-length nude reflection. This should help you see your body objectively. At least it will give you a laugh!

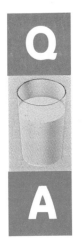

Some diet books insist that you drink 8 glasses of water a day. Others tell you to limit your intake of fluids. What's the big deal about water?

No one should limit their intake of water, say doctors, particularly not people who are lowering their consumption of calories. To do so is dangerous, inviting fatigue at the mild end of the risk scale and serious disease such as kidney stones at the extreme.

Everyone should have the equivalent of 6 to 8 glasses of water a day. Most of us will get a lot of that water from our food. But whatever form it comes in, water is vital for flushing metabolic wastes from our systems. And when we're lowering our intake of calories, we are washing more than the usual amount of waste from our bodies.

You should know, too, that you can't count on your feeling of thirst to tell you when it's time for water. That's what exercise physiologists have discovered. They suggest that, particularly when you're involved in active sports, you should drink as a matter of habit rather than depending on your undependable biological urge. And make it water. Sweetened or so-called metabolic drinks not only contribute unwanted calories but also make it more difficult for your thirsty cells to get the H_2O they need for life.

In addition, water can be an important ally to us when we're working to get leaner. A tall, sparkling glass of water can save you many a calorie. Sometimes the urge to nibble is a disguised form of thirst. And while eating—for instance, a medium apple

(84 percent water) and an ounce of cheddar cheese (37 percent water)—is certainly more entertaining than drinking water, choosing the real thing can save you calories. Often you'll find that your "hunger" will disappear after you've had your water. So make sure you keep an appealing supply of it close at hand, perhaps in an attractive decanter in your refrigerator.

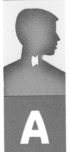

I know people who say they can't lose weight because of a thyroid problem. How common is this? How does the thyroid affect weight anyway?

The thyroid produces a hormone that regulates the rate at which energy is burned in the cells. In almost all people, it functions normally, producing whatever amount of hormone is needed for the energy being burned.

Approximately 3 people in 1,000 have underactive thyroid, experts say. It's a condition that normally is easily diagnosed visually. The victim's fat characteristically appears sickly yellow and the skin is extremely dry. Fortunately, underactive thyroid can usually be treated fairly easily with drugs.

"Most people who say they are overweight because of an underactive thyroid actually have overactive forks," one waggish doctor noted.

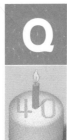

When I was in my twenties, I could easily lose 10 pounds in 2 weeks. Now that I'm in my forties, it's a struggle to lose it in 2 months. Why?

One reason could be that you were probably a lot more active in your twenties. The exercise you did not only burned calories at a faster rate than your present inactivity, but also raised the rate of energy burn-off when you were not exercising. And since you were more active, a higher percentage of your body was muscle. And muscle—even resting muscle—burns calories much faster than fat. Since exercise even dampens the appetite, you may have been eating less though you were doing more.

It's true that the metabolic rate—how fast our cells burn energy—does slow as we age, but not much. The slowdown is as little as 3 percent and certainly no more than 10 percent in the time span from adolescence to middle age, experts say. So the *real* difference between then and now is not due to a slowing of metabolism as much as it is to a slowdown in activity. And that's encouraging news. No matter what your age, you can put the wonderful, calorie-consuming benefits of exercise to work for you.

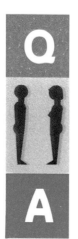

When my husband goes on a diet, he just melts the fat away. Yet, with me, it's always a struggle. I've heard that men can lose weight a lot easier than women. Is it true?

No. The latest word from the scientists is that it's false. Weight loss seems to be one area where there's true equality between the sexes.

A recent study conducted by researchers at the University of Southern California matched men and women by weight before dieting and by factors like age, education and marital status. Both sexes were given instruction in binge control, calorie counting, nutrition, assertiveness, family issues and other helpful topics. The researchers then compared the results obtained over a 13-week period. The conclusion: No real difference in the weight-losing ability of the sexes, either in number of pounds lost (when starting weights were the same) or in percentage of excess lost (when starting weights differed). Women did slightly better than men in the second month, for unknown reasons.

It's no wonder you are confused, though. A lot of bad research has been done in this area. Earlier reports insisted men dieted more successfully than women. Some of this work took no account of starting weights or even of length of time on the diet. Other studies compared people on wholly different programs. Naturally, the results were worthless.

But back to you and your husband. What is true is that if he weighs more than you to start with and you eat the same things in equal portions, he may lose more pounds in the same time. His bigger body needs more calories just to stay even, so he is actually taking a bigger cut than you are. Thus, he drops pounds more quickly. But your proportional loss should be about the same. Of course, calories burned in activity also influence results. Once again, exercise can help both of you lose.

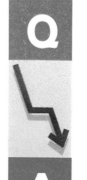

I've been dieting for 2 months, and I was losing a pound a week very steadily. I haven't stopped cutting calories, but I have stopped losing. I'm so frustrated. What can I do?

You are experiencing your body's determination to maintain the status quo. Just as it seeks to maintain a temperature of 98.6°, scientists now believe it has a similar mechanism that seeks to hold your weight steady. Subjected to a regimen of reduced calories, your body reacts by slowing the metabolic rate. It fights to hold on to that fat!

This plateau phenomenon and the discouragement that goes with it seems to be the most common reason people give up on reduced-calorie diets. It's also the main reason that cutting calories alone won't work.

Scientists speculate that this mechanism helped humankind survive periods when the food supply was unreliable. But it's not too helpful to those of us who have found food too plentiful.

What you can do is work some walking into your day, at least 2 walks of not less than 15 minutes each. That'll perk up your metabolic rate and your spirits as well. Again—walking has been found to be an ideal exercise for getting and staying slim. You'll burn nearly as many calories per mile walking briskly as you would jogging.

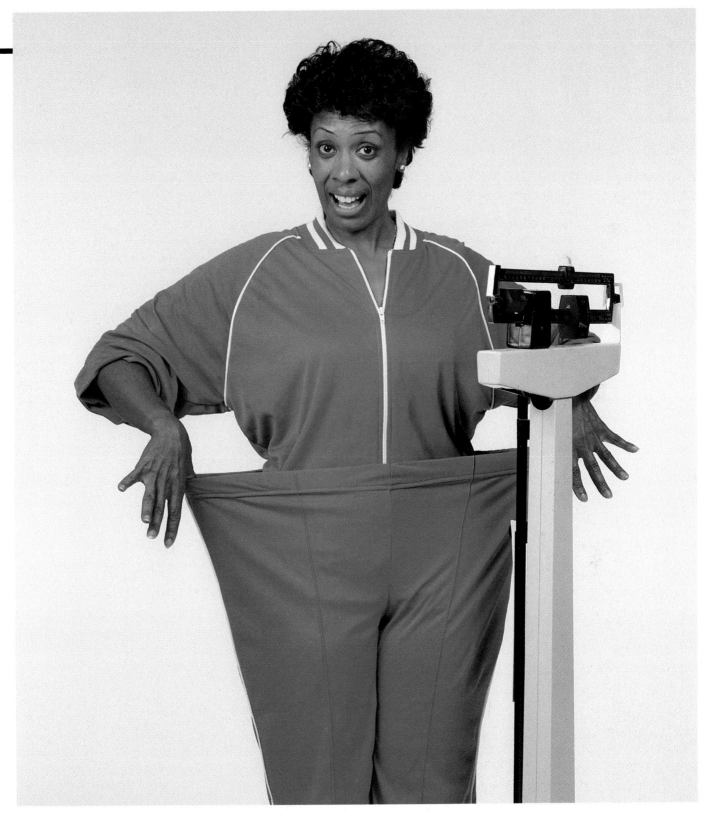

She did it! And you can do it, too. By following the principles outlined in this book, you're well on your way to experiencing the joy of a brand new body—one nourished by healthful food and everyday exercise. And one that will be looking good forever.

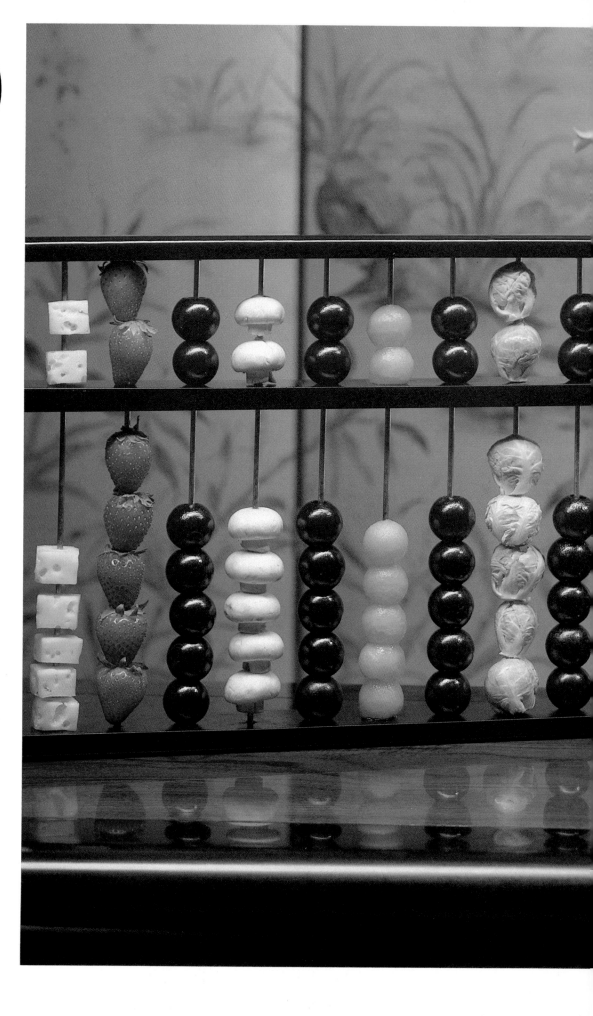

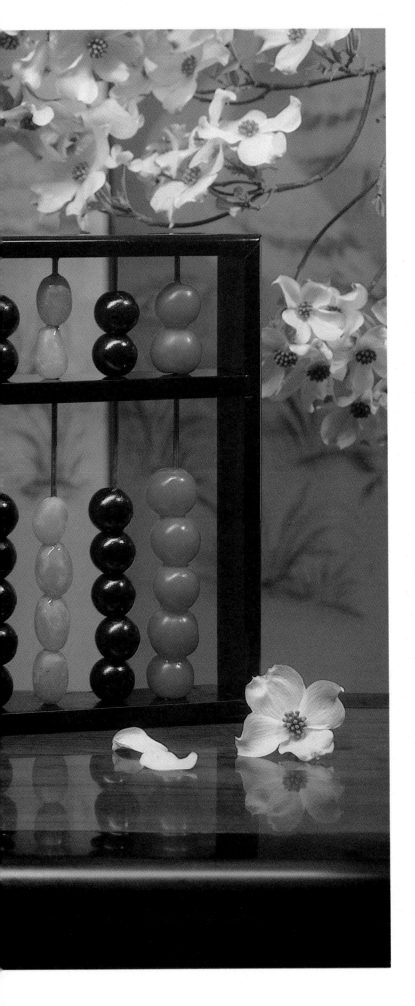

Your Calorie Counter

Become familiar with the caloric value of your favorite foods. It'll help keep your new way of eating on a healthy course.

Y ou're riding high on the positive—healthy eating, feel-good exercise, a new sense of self-worth and well-being. All the wonderful things it takes to control your diet so your diet doesn't control you. Then suddenly the ride stops in front of the salad bar. Your best intentions and 42 selections lie before you— breads, fruits, vegetables, salads galore, not to mention the dessert tray decked out in vanilla, chocolate and strawberry.

How do you know which items you can pile high and which items you shouldn't be piling at all? Let your calorie conscience be your guide.

Hey, what gives? Didn't we just learn that calorie counting doesn't work? That dieting is self-defeating? Indeed we did. But *counting* calories and *being aware* of calories are two different things. After all, it's not always enough to know that fruit is a better alternative for dessert than cake. If it's cake you really want, it's good to know that you'll be a lot better off if you eat a piece of gingerbread rather than a piece of marble cake.

To help raise your calorie consciousness, we're giving you a calorie reference guide that lists values according to food group, with tips on how to use the food in your quest for a healthier diet. And, since we've stressed cutting back on fat throughout this book, we're giving you a fat content guide, too. The figure you see is the *percent of calories* that are fat. For example, if a serving of meat containing 150 calories is 25 percent fat, you'll know that 25 percent of the calories you are eating, *not* 25 percent of the food itself, is fat. It's a figure you should pay close attention to.

Here's to the slim, new you!

Meat, Poultry and Fish

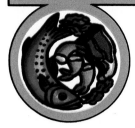

You can get your new eating plan off to a healthy start by decreasing the amount of high-calorie, high-fat red meat that you eat (once or twice a week is often enough) and increasing your intake of lean poultry and fish. This chart and the meat guide on pages 26 and 27 will help you plan your meals wisely. The calorie counts below are for the meat without bone and skin.

Food	Portion	Calories	Percent of Calories from Fat
Bacon			
broiled or fried	3 strips	109	77.5
Canadian-style	2 slices	86	41.1
Bass, striped, fried	3 oz.	168	38.7
Beef			
brisket, choice	3 oz.	189	42.7
brisket, good	3 oz.	169	34.9
chipped, dried	3 oz.	174	24.9
chuck rib roast, choice	3 oz.	212	50.2
chuck rib roast, good	3 oz.	186	42.2
chuck steak, choice	3 oz.	164	33.0
chuck steak, good	3 oz.	152	26.1
club steak, choice	3 oz.	207	48.1
club steak, good	3 oz.	184	39.9
corned	3 oz.	317	73.7
flank steak, choice	3 oz.	167	33.6
flank steak, good	3 oz.	162	31.2
foreshank, choice	3 oz.	156	28.4
foreshank, good	3 oz.	150	24.6
heart	3 oz.	160	28.2
heel of round, choice	3 oz.	153	28.6
heel of round, good	3 oz.	148	25.9
hindshank, choice	3 oz.	156	28.9
hindshank, good	3 oz.	150	24.6
ground, regular	3 oz.	243	64.0
ground, lean	3 oz.	186	46.5
liver, fried	3 oz.	195	41.6
porterhouse steak, choice	3 oz.	190	42.3
porterhouse steak, good	3 oz.	167	32.5
round steak, choice	3 oz.	162	30.2
round steak, good	3 oz.	149	22.2
rump roast, choice	3 oz.	177	40.3
rump roast, good	3 oz.	162	33.7
sirloin steak, choice	3 oz.	204	47.0
sirloin steak, good	3 oz.	178	37.1
chuck cubes, for stew	3 oz.	183	40.0
T-bone steak, choice	3 oz.	190	41.7
T-bone steak, good	3 oz.	169	33.1
tongue	3 oz.	208	60.7
Bluefish, baked with butter	3 oz.	135	26.7
Bologna			
beef	1 oz.	89	81.5
lebanon	1 oz.	64	59.3
pork	1 oz.	70	72.5
turkey	1 oz.	57	68.2
Bratwurst	1 oz.	85	77.8
Braunschweiger	1 oz.	102	80.5
Chicken			
back	3 oz.	204	49.4
breast	3 oz.	140	19.5
drumstick	3 oz.	147	29.6
giblets	3 oz.	134	27.4
leg	3 oz.	163	39.7
liver	3 oz.	133	31.4
thigh	3 oz.	178	46.8
wing	3 oz.	174	35.9
Chicken liver pâté	3 oz.	171	58.7
Chicken roll, light meat	1 oz.	45	41.9

Food	Portion	Calories	Percent of Calories from Fat
Clams			
cherrystones	6	84	9.7
chowders	6	156	10.2
littlenecks	6	67	9.7
Cod, broiled with butter	3 oz.	144	28.2
Crab			
king, steamed	3 oz.	79	18.2
deviled	3 oz.	160	45.2
imperial	3 oz.	125	46.6
Duck, domesticated	3 oz.	171	50.2
Fish cakes	5 sm.	103	42.0
Flounder, baked with butter	3 oz.	171	36.4
Frankfurter			
beef	1	184	82.2
chicken	1	116	68.1
turkey	1	102	70.4
Goose, domesticated	3 oz.	202	48.0
Haddock, breaded, fried	3 oz.	141	34.5
Halibut, broiled with butter	3 oz.	144	37.6
Ham			
cured	3 oz.	140	41.9
fresh	3 oz.	187	45.2
picnic, cured	3 oz.	251	37.2
picnic, fresh	3 oz.	194	49.9
sliced	1 oz.	52	52.0
Ham salad spread	1 oz.	61	65.1
Herring			
plain	3 oz.	177	59.0
pickled	3 oz.	189	61.6
smoked, kippered	3 oz.	179	55.1
Knockwurst	3 oz.	261	81.6
Lamb			
leg	3 oz.	158	34.3
loin chops	3 oz.	160	36.2
rib chops	3 oz.	180	45.1
shoulder	3 oz.	170	41.6
Liverwurst	3 oz.	279	78.5
Lobster			
broiled	3 oz.	81	14.2
Newburg	½ cup	243	49.3
Mackerel, broiled with butter	3 oz.	201	60.6
Mussels	6	25	21.0
Ocean perch, breaded, fried	3 oz.	195	50.9
Oysters, fried	6	163	51.7
Pepperoni	1 oz.	139	80.8
Pork			
Blade roll, cured	3 oz.	244	73.7
Boston blade, fresh	3 oz.	218	59.2
loin chops	3 oz.	232	48.3
spareribs	3 oz.	545	68.7
Rockfish, steamed	3 oz.	90	21.0
Salami			
beef, cooked	1 oz.	72	71.4
beef and pork	1 oz.	71	72.4
pork, hard	1 oz.	115	74.7
Salmon			
chinook	3 oz.	179	60.1

Food	Portion	Calories	Percent of Calories from Fat
pink	3 oz.	120	37.8
smoked	3 oz.	150	46.9
red sockeye	3 oz.	145	49.2
steak, broiled with butter	3 oz.	156	36.4
Sardines	3 oz.	175	46.4
Sausage			
Italian	1	268	71.8
link, smoked	3 oz.	331	73.5
Polish	3 oz.	276	79.8
Vienna	3 oz.	239	80.8
Scallops	6	67	11.4
Shad, baked with butter	3 oz.	170	53.1
Shrimp			
canned	6 med.	22	9.8
french fried	6 med.	44	43.7
Swordfish, broiled with butter	3 oz.	138	31.4
Tilefish	3 oz.	117	23.1
Trout, steamed	3 oz.	115	30.1
Tuna			
canned, oil	3 oz.	245	64.2
canned, water	3 oz.	108	5.6
Turkey			
breast	3 oz.	115	4.9
giblets	3 oz.	142	27.4
leg	3 oz.	135	21.5
wing	3 oz.	139	19.1
Turkey roll, light meat	1 oz.	42	44.0
Veal			
chuck cubes, for stew	3 oz.	200	49.1
cutlet	3 oz.	185	43.9
loin	3 oz.	199	51.7
plate, breast of veal	3 oz.	256	63.1
rib roast	3 oz.	230	54.9
round roast	3 oz.	184	46.1

Vegetables and Legumes

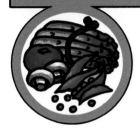

You can't go wrong increasing your intake of these foods— at every meal. They contain the complex carbohydrates and fiber you need for a healthy eating program. And don't forget this food group when the hunger pangs hit, either. Raw vegetables make great snack foods.

Food	Portion	Calories	Percent of Calories from Fat
Artichoke	1 globe	32	5.4
Asparagus	4 med. spears	12	6.7
Bamboo shoots	¼ cup	10	9.8
Beans			
black, dried	¼ cup	170	3.7
Great Northern	½ cup	106	4.3
green, French-style	½ cup	17	2.4
green, snap	½ cup	16	8.4
kidney	½ cup	109	3.5
lima	½ cup	95	4.0
mung, sprouted	½ cup	18	7.4
navy	½ cup	112	4.1
pinto, dried	¼ cup	166	2.9
yellow	½ cup	14	9.3
Beets, diced or sliced	½ cup	27	3.0
Beet greens			
cooked	½ cup	13	10.0
raw	1 cup	13	10.8
Broccoli, raw	1 med. stalk	48	8.1
Brussels sprouts	4	30	8.4
Cabbage			
Chinese, raw	½ cup	6	7.6
raw	½ cup	11	7.6
red, raw	½ cup	14	6.0
Carrots			
cooked	½ cup	23	5.6
raw	1 med.	30	2.8
Cauliflower, cooked	½ cup	14	9.0
Celery, chopped, raw	½ cup	10	4.2
Chick-peas, dried	¼ cup	180	11.2
Chicory	1 cup	14	6.0
Chowchow, sweet	¼ cup	71	6.5
Coleslaw	½ cup	60	66.8
Collards, cooked	½ cup	32	17.3
Corn			
cooked, on the cob	1 ear	70	9.6
cream style	½ cup	93	4.2
Cucumbers, sliced	½ cup	8	5.2
Dandelion greens, cooked	½ cup	18	14.3
Eggplant	½ cup	19	8.8
Endive	1 cup	10	8.4
Kale, cooked	½ cup	22	15.6
Kohlrabi	½ cup	20	4.2
Lentils			
dried	¼ cup	162	2.7
red, dried	¼ cup	145	2.6
Lettuce			
Bibb	1 cup	8	10.5
iceberg	1 cup	7	12.0
looseleaf	1 cup	10	16.7
romaine	1 cup	10	16.7
Mixed vegetables	½ cup	58	3.6
Mushrooms, raw	½ cup	10	8.4
Mustard greens, cooked	½ cup	16	15.7
Mustard spinach, cooked	½ cup	15	11.5
Okra	½ cup	23	9.1
Onions			
cooked	¼ cup	15	2.7
raw	¼ cup	16	2.6
Parsley, dried	1 tsp.	1	8.4
Parsnips	½ cup	51	6.6
Peas			
and carrots, mixed	½ cup	41	4.8
blackeye	½ cup	89	6.1
green	½ cup	57	4.4
sweet green	½ cup	59	4.6
Peppers			
green, raw	1 med.	36	7.0
sweet red, raw	1 med.	51	8.2
Pickles			
dill	1 med.	7	12.0

Food	Portion	Calories	Percent of Calories from Fat
sweet gherkin	1 lg.	51	1.6
Potatoes			
baked	1 med.	145	1.2
boiled with skin	1 med.	173	1.0
french fried	10 strips	137	40.3
hashed brown	½ cup	178	42.7
mashed	½ cup	69	9.2
salad	½ cup	182	53.0
Pumpkin, canned	½ cup	40	7.4
Radishes	3 lg.	4	6.0
Rutabaga	½ cup	30	2.8
Sauerkraut	½ cup	25	8.4
Scallions	¼ cup	11	3.7
Shallots	¼ cup	28	trace
Soybeans, cooked	½ cup	117	36.8
Spinach			
cooked	½ cup	21	10.2
raw	1 cup	14	12.0

Food	Portion	Calories	Percent of Calories from Fat
Squash			
acorn, mashed	½ cup	57	1.5
butternut, mashed	½ cup	70	1.2
hubbard, mashed	½ cup	52	6.5
yellow	½ cup	14	12.4
Succotash	½ cup	73	7.1
Sweet potatoes			
baked	1	161	3.1
candied	1	245	16.6
Swiss chard, cooked	½ cup	16	10.5
Tofu	3 oz.	61	48.7
Tomatoes			
cooked	½ cup	32	6.6
raw	1 med.	27	6.2
Turnips, cooked	½ cup	18	7.0
Turnip greens, cooked	½ cup	15	8.7
Watercress	¼ cup	2	12.0
Zucchini, raw	½ cup	11	3.8

Fruits

Try to make a piece of fruit a part of every meal. But if you're really watching calories, you might want to be a bit discriminating in the fruits you select. "Going bananas"— or figs or avocados or raisins—can add on the calories real fast! Naturally, we suggest you stick with fresh fruit whenever possible.

Food	Portion	Calories	Percent of Calories from Fat
Apples			
canned, sweetened, sliced	½ cup	68	6.2
cooked	½ cup	46	5.8
dried	½ cup	105	1.1
fresh	1	81	5.1
Applesauce			
canned, sweetened	½ cup	97	2.1
canned, unsweetened	½ cup	53	0.9
Apricots			
canned, heavy syrup	½ cup	107	0.8
canned, juice pack	½ cup	60	0.6
canned, light syrup	½ cup	80	0.6
canned, water pack	½ cup	33	5.0
dehydrated	½ cup	192	1.6
dried	½ cup	155	1.6
fresh	3	51	6.7
Avocado	1	324	79.5
Bananas			
dehydrated	½ cup	173	4.4
fresh	1	105	4.4
Blackberries			
canned, heavy syrup	½ cup	118	1.3
fresh	½ cup	37	6.3
frozen, unsweetened	½ cup	49	5.6
Blueberries			
canned, heavy syrup	½ cup	112	3.2
fresh	½ cup	41	5.6
frozen, sweetened	½ cup	94	1.4
frozen, unsweetened	½ cup	39	10.6
Boysenberries			
canned, heavy syrup	½ cup	113	1.1
frozen, unsweetened	½ cup	33	4.4
Cantaloupe	¼ melon	47	6.6
Casaba	⅛ melon	54	3.1
Cherries			
sour, red	½ cup	39	5.1

Food	Portion	Calories	Percent of Calories from Fat
sour, canned, heavy syrup	½ cup	116	0.9
sour, canned, light syrup	½ cup	94	1.1
sour, canned, water pack	½ cup	43	2.3
sour, frozen, unsweetened	½ cup	36	7.9
sweet	½ cup	52	11.2
sweet, canned, heavy syrup	½ cup	107	1.5
sweet, canned, juice pack	½ cup	68	0.3
sweet, canned, light syrup	½ cup	85	1.9
sweet, canned, water pack	½ cup	57	2.3
sweet, frozen, sweetened	½ cup	116	1.2
Cranberries	½ cup	23	3.5
Cranberry sauce, canned, sweetened	½ cup	209	0.8
Cranberry-orange relish, canned	½ cup	246	0.5
Currants, black	¼ cup	18	5.3
Dates, chopped	¼ cup	122	1.4
Elderberries	½ cup	53	5.8
Figs			
canned, heavy syrup	¼ cup	57	1.0
canned, light syrup	¼ cup	43	1.3
canned, water pack	¼ cup	33	1.6
dried	¼ cup	127	3.8
fresh	2 med.	74	3.4
Fruit cocktail			
canned, heavy syrup	½ cup	93	0.8
canned, juice pack	½ cup	56	0.3
canned, light syrup	½ cup	72	1.0
canned, water pack	½ cup	40	1.3
Gooseberries			
canned, light syrup	½ cup	93	2.3
fresh	½ cup	34	10.9
Grapefruit			
pink	½	37	2.7
white	½	39	2.6

Food	Portion	Calories	Percent of Calories from Fat
Grapes	10	15	4.5
Guava	½ cup	42	10.0
Honeydew	⅛ melon	58	2.4
Kiwi fruit	1 med.	46	6.2
Kumquats	3	36	1.4
Lemon	1 wedge	3	8.4
Lime	1 wedge	3	5.4
Loganberries, frozen	½ cup	40	4.8
Mango	½	68	3.5
Mixed fruit			
canned, heavy syrup	½ cup	92	1.2
frozen, sweetened	½ cup	123	1.6
Mulberries	¼ cup	15	7.5
Nectarine	1	67	7.7
Oranges			
navel	1	65	1.7
Valencia	1	59	5.1
Papaya	½	59	3.1
Passion-fruit	1	18	6.0
Peaches			
canned, heavy syrup	½ cup	95	1.1
canned, juice pack	½ cup	55	0.6
canned, light syrup	½ cup	68	0.5
canned, water pack	½ cup	29	2.0
dehydrated	½ cup	188	2.7
fresh	1	37	1.8
Pears			
canned, heavy syrup	½ cup	94	1.5
canned, juice pack	½ cup	62	1.1
canned, light syrup	½ cup	72	0.5
canned, water pack	½ cup	36	0.8
dried	½ cup	236	2.0
fresh	1	98	5.6
Persimmon	1	32	2.6
Pineapple			
canned, heavy syrup	½ cup	100	1.2

Food	Portion	Calories	Percent of Calories from Fat
canned, juice pack	½ cup	75	1.2
canned, light syrup	½ cup	66	1.9
canned, water pack	½ cup	40	2.4
fresh	1 slice (3½″ × ¾″)	42	7.2
Plums	3	108	9.5
Pomegranate	1	104	3.7
Prickly pear	1	42	10.6
Prunes			
canned, heavy syrup	5	90	1.6
dried, cooked, sweetened	½ cup	147	1.5
dried, cooked, unsweetened	½ cup	113	1.8
Quince	1	53	1.4
Raisins			
golden, seedless	¼ cup	125	1.3
seedless	¼ cup	124	1.3
Raspberries			
fresh	¼ cup	15	9.3
red, canned, heavy syrup	¼ cup	59	1.1
red, frozen, sweetened	¼ cup	64	1.3
Rhubarb			
fresh, diced	½ cup	13	7.7
frozen, cooked, sweetened	½ cup	139	0.4
frozen, uncooked	½ cup	14	4.8
Strawberries			
canned, heavy syrup	¼ cup	59	2.4
fresh	¼ cup	11	10.2
frozen, unsweetened	¼ cup	13	2.6
sliced, frozen, sweetened	¼ cup	61	1.1
Tangerines			
canned, juice pack	½ cup	46	0.5
canned, light syrup	½ cup	76	1.4
fresh	1	37	3.6
Watermelon	1 slice (10″ × 1″)	152	11.3

Breads, Cereals and Grains

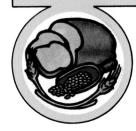

Go for the whole grains if you want this food group to work for you. Put a portion or two into your diet every day—especially at breakfast. But check for the fat in some of the cereals—it has a tendency to sneak up on you.

Food	Portion	Calories	Percent of Calories from Fat
All-Bran	½ cup	107	5.9
Biscuits			
baking powder	1	103	39.0
from mix	1	91	23.9
Bran Buds	½ cup	109	7.7
Bran Chex	½ cup	78	7.5
Bread crumbs			
dry, grated	1 cup	392	9.8
white	1 cup	124	11.5
Bread sticks	2	38	6.5
Cheerios	½ cup	44	13.6
Corn Bran	½ cup	62	8.9
Corn Chex	½ cup	56	0.8
Cornflakes	½ cup	52	0.8
Corn grits	½ cup	73	2.9
Cornbread, whole ground	1 piece	161	29.1
Cornmeal, whole ground	¼ cup	108	9.3

Food	Portion	Calories	Percent of Calories from Fat
Cracked wheat bread	1 slice	66	7.6
Cracklin' Bran	½ cup	115	33.4
Cream of Wheat	½ cup	67	3.1
Crispy Wheats 'n Raisins	½ cup	75	3.9
Farina	½ cup	58	1.4
Flour			
lima bean	¼ cup	108	3.5
buckwheat, dark	¼ cup	82	6.4
buckwheat, light	¼ cup	85	3.0
carob	¼ cup	63	6.6
corn	¼ cup	108	5.8
peanut, defatted	¼ cup	56	20.6
rye, dark	¼ cup	105	6.6
rye, light	¼ cup	79	2.4
rye, medium	¼ cup	77	4.1
soybean, defatted	¼ cup	82	2.3
white	¼ cup	105	2.4
whole wheat	¼ cup	100	5.0

Food	Portion	Calories	Percent of Calories from Fat
Fortified Oat Flakes	½ cup	89	3.3
40% bran flakes	½ cup	73	4.2
French bread	1 slice	102	9.0
Granola, homemade	½ cup	298	47.8
Grape-Nuts	½ cup	202	0.8
Heartland Natural Cereal, plain	½ cup	250	30.5
Italian bread	1 slice	83	2.0
Life	½ cup	81	4.1
Macaroni, elbows and shells, cooked	1 cup	192	3.1
Most	½ cup	88	2.9
Muffins			
blueberry	1	112	27.7
bran	1	104	31.4
cornmeal, whole ground	1	115	29.8
plain	1	118	28.4
Nature Valley Granola	½ cup	252	33.5
Noodles, egg, cooked	1 cup	200	10.0
Nutri-Grain			
barley	½ cup	77	1.6
corn	½ cup	80	5.2
rye	½ cup	72	1.7
wheat	½ cup	79	2.6
Oatmeal	½ cup	73	13.9
100% Bran	½ cup	89	15.5
100% Natural Cereal, plain	½ cup	245	39.4
Pancakes			
buckwheat	1	146	37.8
plain or buttermilk	1	164	27.0
Pita bread, whole wheat	1 pocket	128	11.0
Product 19	½ cup	63	1.3
Puffed rice	½ cup	28	1.5
Puffed wheat	½ cup	22	1.9

Food	Portion	Calories	Percent of Calories from Fat
Pumpernickel bread	1 slice	79	4.2
Raisin bran	½ cup	84	3.7
Raisin bread	1 slice	66	8.9
Ralston	½ cup	67	5.0
Rice			
brown, long grain, cooked	½ cup	116	4.3
white, long grain, cooked	½ cup	112	0.8
Rice Chex	½ cup	50	0.7
Rice Krispies	½ cup	56	1.5
Rolls			
brown-and-serve	1	84	18.9
frankfurter or hamburger	1	119	15.5
hard, kaiser	1	156	8.6
hoagie	1	392	8.8
Rye bread	1 slice	61	4.1
Rye wafers, whole grain	1	22	3.0
Shredded wheat	2 lg.	166	3.0
Spaghetti, cooked "al dente" (firm)	1 cup	192	3.1
Special K	½ cup	42	0.8
Total	½ cup	58	5.1
Waffle	1 section	138	32.1
Wheat 'n Raisin Chex	½ cup	93	1.8
Wheat Chex	½ cup	85	5.5
Wheat germ, toasted, plain	½ cup	216	23.5
Wheatena	½ cup	68	6.8
Wheaties	½ cup	51	4.1
White bread			
firm crumb	1 slice	74	11.3
soft crumb	1 slice	76	9.9
Whole wheat bread			
firm crumb	1 slice	61	11.0
soft crumb	1 slice	67	8.7

Desserts and Snacks

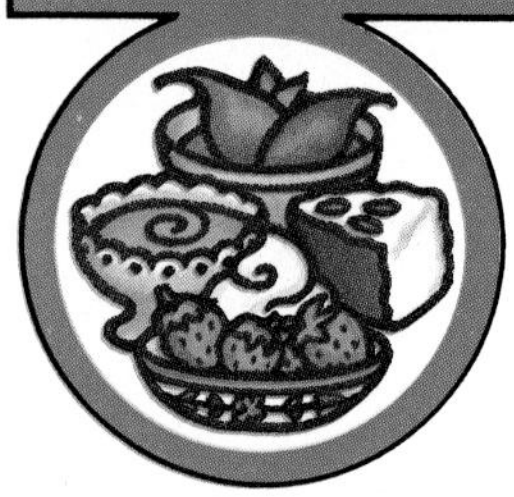

You can't be expected to say no to cookies, candy, cakes and other snacks and goodies *all* the time. This list should help keep you from going overboard on those occasional times when you do say yes.

Food	Portion	Calories	Percent of Calories from Fat
Apple brown betty	½ cup	163	19.3
Brownie, with nuts	1	97	54.4
Cakes*			
angel food	1 slice	137	0.6
caramel, with icing, 2-layer	1 slice	398	32.6
coffee	1 slice (⅙ cake)	232	24.9
devil's food, with chocolate icing	1 slice	312	30.3
devil's food, with white icing	1 slice	362	33.1
fruit cake, dark	1 slice (1/30 loaf)	57	33.8
fruit cake, light	1 slice (1/30 loaf)	58	36.1
gingerbread	1 slice (⅑ cake)	174	20.7
marble, with white icing	1 slice	288	22.1

*Unless otherwise noted, 1 slice equals 1/12 cake.

Food	Portion	Calories	Percent of Calories from Fat
pound	1 slice	142	52.5
sponge	1 slice	196	16.2
white, with chocolate icing	1 slice	333	25.6
white, with coconut icing	1 slice	386	29.9
white, without icing	1 slice	264	35.7
yellow, with chocolate icing	1 slice	310	28.1
yellow, without icing	1 slice	263	29.3
Candy			
butterscotch	1 oz.	113	8.0
chocolate caramel	1 oz.	113	23.1
chocolate, bittersweet	1 oz.	135	70.1
chocolate, milk	1 oz.	147	52.4
chocolate, milk, with peanuts	1 oz.	154	58.7
chocolate, semisweet	1 oz.	144	58.7
chocolate-coated almonds	1 oz.	161	64.5
chocolate-coated, chocolate fudge center	1 oz.	122	30.9

Food	Portion	Calories	Percent of Calories from Fat
chocolate-coated, coconut center	1 oz.	124	33.8
chocolate-coated fudge, caramel and peanuts	1 oz.	123	34.7
chocolate-coated nougat and caramel	1 oz.	118	27.7
chocolate-coated raisins	1 oz.	120	33.5
chocolate-coated vanilla creams	1 oz.	123	32.7
fudge, chocolate	1 oz.	113	25.9
fudge, vanilla	1 oz.	113	23.0
gumdrops	1 oz.	98	1.8
hard	1 oz.	109	2.5
jelly beans	1 oz.	104	0.9
marshmallow	1 lg.	23	trace
peanut brittle	1 oz.	119	21.9
Chocolate syrup	1 tbsp.	46	7.3
Cookies			
chocolate chip	4	206	48.8
fig bars	4	200	13.0
ladyfingers	4	158	18.0
macaroons	4	362	40.7
molasses	4	548	20.8
oatmeal with raisins	4	235	28.5
sandwich	4	198	38.0
shortbread	4	150	38.7
Crackers			
animal	10	112	17.9
butter	10	151	32.7
cheese	10	52	37.0
graham, plain	1 lg.	55	19.8
graham, sugar honey	1 lg.	58	23.1
oyster	10	33	25.4
saltine	10	123	23.1
sandwich, cheese and peanut butter	6	209	40.8
soda	10	125	24.8
Cream puff	1	303	50.0
Custard, baked	½ cup	153	42.1
Doughnut, plain	1	164	39.8
Eclair	1	239	47.6
Gelatin	½ cup	71	0

Food	Portion	Calories	Percent of Calories from Fat
Ice cream			
hardened, vanilla	1 cup	269	46.8
soft serve, French vanilla	1 cup	377	52.5
Ice milk			
hardened, vanilla	1 cup	184	26.9
soft serve, vanilla	1 cup	223	18.2
Nuts			
almonds, dry, whole	¼ cup	212	75.9
almonds, roasted, salted	¼ cup	246	77.1
Brazil nuts, whole	¼ cup	229	85.6
cashews, whole	¼ cup	196	68.2
chestnuts	½ cup	155	6.5
peanuts, roasted, salted	¼ cup	211	71.3
pecans, halves	¼ cup	186	86.7
walnuts	¼ cup	196	79.0
Pies†			
apple	1 slice	302	36.3
banana custard	1 slice	252	35.2
blackberry	1 slice	287	37.9
blueberry	1 slice	286	37.2
Boston cream	1 slice	311	26.1
cherry	1 slice	308	36.1
coconut custard	1 slice	268	44.7
lemon meringue	1 slice	268	33.4
pecan	1 slice	431	45.8
pumpkin	1 slice	241	44.5
Popcorn			
oil and salt added	1 cup	41	40.8
plain	1 cup	23	10.9
sugar-coated	1 cup	134	7.5
Potato chips	10	114	58.7
Pretzels			
rod	1	55	9.1
twisted	1	62	9.5
Pudding			
chocolate	½ cup	161	21.3
cottage, without sauce	1 slice	186	27.5
rice, with raisins	½ cup	194	18.6
Sherbet, orange	1 cup	270	12.4
Sunflower seeds	¼ cup	203	70.7
Tapioca	½ cup	111	33.4

†One slice equals ⅛ pie.

Condiments

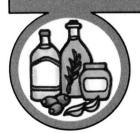

A sprinkling of Worcestershire, a dab of mustard—sometimes the things you add as flavorings don't register as a part of your caloric buildup. But some items you use as condiments. most notoriously oils and dressings, can pack a lot of calories into a tablespoon. Use them wisely.

Food	Portion	Calories	Percent of Calories from Fat
Cocoa powder	4 heaping tsp.	106	6.4
Croutons	¼ cup	28	8.3
Horseradish	1 tsp.	2	trace
Ketchup	1 tsp.	5	5.6
Mayonnaise	1 tbsp.	99	98.3
Mustard			
brown	1 tsp.	5	54.0
yellow	1 tsp.	4	45.0

Food	Portion	Calories	Percent of Calories from Fat
Oil			
olive	1 tbsp.	119	100.0
safflower	1 tbsp.	120	100.0
Pickle relish	1 tsp.	7	4.3
Salad dressings			
blue cheese	1 tbsp.	77	91.7
French	1 tbsp.	67	84.4
Italian	1 tbsp.	69	91.4
Russian	1 tbsp.	76	90.7
Thousand Island	1 tbsp.	59	84.0

Food	Portion	Calories	Percent of Calories from Fat
Sauces			
barbecue	1 tsp.	4	20.3
chili	1 tsp.	5	2.8
cocktail, seafood	1 tbsp.	22	trace
soy	1 tsp.	4	0

Food	Portion	Calories	Percent of Calories from Fat
sweet-and-sour	1 tsp.	6	0.2
teriyaki	1 tsp.	3	5.9
Worcestershire	1 tbsp.	13	0
Tomato paste	¼ cup	54	3.9
Vinegar, cider	1 tbsp.	2	0

Dairy Products

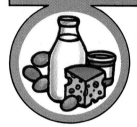

More than any other food group, milk and its products are major dietary sources of calcium—contributing some 72 percent to the American food supply. This alone should be enough to convince you to include dairy products, particularly milk and cheese, in your daily diet. The negative side of the coin is that many dairy products are high in fat and should be used sparingly.

Food	Portion	Calories	Percent of Calories from Fat
Butter	1 tbsp.	102	99.1
Cheese*			
caraway	1 oz.	107	68.0
Cheshire	1 oz.	110	69.4
Colby	1 oz.	112	71.4
Edam	1 oz.	101	68.6
Fontina	1 oz.	110	70.6
Gouda	1 oz.	101	67.7
Gruyere	1 oz.	117	68.9
Monterey	1 oz.	106	71.1
Muenster	1 oz.	104	72.0
Port du Salut	1 oz.	100	70.3
Provolone	1 oz.	100	66.4
Romano	1 oz.	110	61.1
Cheese spread	1 oz.	82	64.5
Cream			
light	1 tbsp.	29	87.9
whipping, heavy	1 tbsp.	52	93.8
whipping, light	1 tbsp.	44	92.7

*Additional cheeses are listed on page 29.

Food	Portion	Calories	Percent of Calories from Fat
Egg	1 lg.	79	63.7
Half-and-half	1 tbsp.	20	75.6
Margarine	1 tsp.	34	98.2
Milk			
buttermilk	1 cup	99	19.2
chocolate	1 cup	208	35.8
dry, nonfat	¼ cup	109	1.9
dry, whole	¼ cup	159	47.3
evaporated	¼ cup	85	49.3
low fat, 1%	1 cup	102	22.3
low fat, 2%	1 cup	121	34.0
skim	1 cup	86	4.5
whole, 3.3% fat	1 cup	150	47.8
Sour cream	1 tbsp.	26	85.2
Yogurt			
low fat, fruit varieties	1 cup	225	10.2
low fat, plain	1 cup	144	21.5
skim milk, plain	1 cup	127	2.8
whole milk, plain	1 cup	139	46.7

Soups, Sauces and Gravies

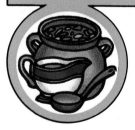

Soup—the noncreamy variety—is great for filling you up without filling you out. In fact, studies have proven soups are a real asset to the weight watcher. Make an effort to keep away from sauces and gravies laden with fat.

Food	Portion	Calories	Percent of Calories from Fat
Asparagus soup, cream of, prepared with milk	1 cup	161	44.7
Au jus gravy	1 tbsp.	2	11.4
Bean soup			
black	1 cup	116	11.5
with bacon	1 cup	173	30.9
Bearnaise sauce	1 tbsp.	44	81.8
Beef broth	1 cup	16	29.8

Food	Portion	Calories	Percent of Calories from Fat
Beef gravy	1 tbsp.	8	39.8
Beef noodle soup	1 cup	84	32.6
Celery soup, cream of, prepared with milk	1 cup	165	51.6
Cheese sauce	1 tbsp.	19	49.0
Cheese soup, prepared with milk	1 cup	230	57.0
Chicken broth	1 cup	39	32.1

Food	Portion	Calories	Percent of Calories from Fat
Chicken gravy	1 tbsp.	12	64.1
Chicken soup			
chunky	1 cup	178	33.5
with noodles	1 cup	75	29.1
Clam chowder			
Manhattan	1 cup	78	26.7
New England, prepared			
with milk	1 cup	163	36.0
Consomme	1 cup	29	0
Crab soup	1 cup	76	17.9
Curry sauce	1 tbsp.	17	45.7
Gazpacho	1 cup	57	35.4
Hollandaise sauce, prepared			
with eggs and butter	1 tbsp.	84	85.0
Lentil soup, with ham	1 cup	140	17.9
Minestrone soup	1 cup	83	27.2
Mushroom sauce	1 tbsp.	14	38.0
Mushroom soup, cream of,			
prepared with milk	1 cup	203	58.9
Onion soup	1 cup	57	27.2
Oyster stew, prepared			
with milk	1 cup	134	52.7
Pea soup			
green, prepared with water	1 cup	164	15.8
split, with ham	1 cup	189	21.0
Potato soup, cream of,			
prepared with milk	1 cup	148	38.4
Scotch broth	1 cup	80	29.5
Shrimp soup, cream of,			
prepared with milk	1 cup	165	50.1
Sour cream sauce	1 tbsp.	32	49.9
Spaghetti sauce			
plain	1 tbsp.	42	3.0
with mushrooms	1 tbsp.	45	25.5
Stroganoff sauce	1 tbsp.	17	33.2
Tomato bisque, prepared			
with water	1 cup	123	18.4
Tomato soup			
prepared with water	1 cup	86	19.9
with rice	1 cup	120	20.2
Turkey gravy	1 tbsp.	8	36.5
Turkey soup			
with noodles	1 cup	69	25.7
with vegetables	1 cup	74	36.7
Vegetable soup			
with beef	1 cup	79	21.6
vegetarian	1 cup	72	23.9
White sauce	1 tbsp.	15	46.9

Beverages

Because they slide so easily down the throat, it's sometimes easy to let the caloric value of some of your favorite beverages — particularly the alcoholic variety — slip your mind. Our advice — don't! Keep track of them, just as you would any food.

Food	Portion	Calories	Percent of Calories from Fat
Ale	12 oz.	147	trace
Apple cider	½ cup	59	trace
Apple juice	½ cup	58	2.0
Apricot nectar	½ cup	71	1.3
Beer	12 oz.	151	0
Bitter lemon	6 oz.	96	0
Brandy	3 oz.	207	0
Club soda	6 oz.	0	0
Coffee, brewed	1 cup	4	3.0
Colas			
with sugar	12 oz.	159	0
sugar free	12 oz.	2	0
Cranberry juice cocktail	1 cup	147	0.7
Cream soda	12 oz.	156	0
Daiquiri	3½ oz.	122	0
Eggnog	1 cup	342	48.8
Fruit punch drink	1 cup	132	0.2
Gin, rum, vodka, whiskey			
80 proof	1½ oz.	97	0
100 proof	1½ oz.	124	0
Ginger ale	12 oz.	113	0
Grapefruit juice	½ cup	48	2.2
Lemonade	1 cup	107	trace
Manhattan	3¼ oz.	233	0
Martini	2½ oz.	152	0
Milk shake, chocolate	1	356	20.0
Mineral water	8 oz.	0	0
Orange juice	½ cup	56	3.8
Pineapple juice			
canned	½ cup	70	1.2
frozen, diluted	½ cup	65	0.5
Peach nectar	½ cup	67	0.3
Pear nectar	½ cup	75	0.2
Prune juice	½ cup	91	0.4
Root beer	12 oz.	163	0
Sodas, fruit-flavored			
with sugar	12 oz.	166	0
sugar free	12 oz.	3	0
Tea			
brewed	1 cup	0	0
iced, instant, sweetened	1 cup	86	0.7
Tomato juice cocktail	1 cup	51	3.3
Tonic water	12 oz.	132	0
Whiskey sour	3½ oz.	184	0
Wines			
champagne	3½ oz.	71	0
dessert, sweet	3½ oz.	153	0
port	3 oz.	134	0
red table	3½ oz.	76	0
sherry	3½ oz.	147	0
vermouth, dry	3½ oz.	105	0
vermouth, sweet	3½ oz.	184	0
white table	3½ oz.	80	0

Source Notes

Chapter 1

Page 2

"Average Body Weights since 1850" adapted from "Obesity: The American Disease" by Theodore B. Van Itallie, M.D., *Food Technology*, December, 1979
and
NHANES II studies conducted by the National Center for Health Statistics.

Page 14

"Desirable Weights for Men" adapted from (1959) "Desirable Weights for Men and Women," *Statistical Bulletin*, October, 1977 (New York: Metropolitan Life Insurance Co.)
and
"1983 Height and Weight Tables," Metropolitan Life Insurance Co. news release, March 1, 1983. Reprinted by permission of Metropolitan Life Insurance Co.

Page 15

"Desirable Weights for Women" adapted from (1959) "Desirable Weights for Men And Women," *Statistical Bulletin*, October, 1977 (New York: Metropolitan Life Insurance Co.)
and
"1983 Height And Weight Tables," Metropolitan Life Insurance Co. news release, March 1, 1983. Reprinted by permission of Metropolitan Life Insurance Co.

Chapter 2

Page 26

"The Choicest Cuts" adapted from *Composition of Foods: Poultry Products*, Agriculture Handbook No. 8-5, by Consumer and Food Economics Institute (Washington, D.C.: Science and Education Administration, U.S. Department of Agriculture, 1979)
and
Nutritive Value of American Foods in Common Units, Agriculture Handbook No. 456, by Catherine F. Adams (Washington, D.C.: Agricultural Research Service, U.S. Department of Agriculture, 1975)
and
Proximate Composition of Beef from Carcass to Cooked Meat: Method of Derivation and Tables of Values, Home Economics Research Report No. 31, by Consumer and Food Economics Division (Washington, D.C.: Agricultural Research Service, U.S. Department of Agriculture, 1972).

Page 29

"Calories at a Glance" adapted from *Composition of Foods: Dairy and Egg Products*, Agriculture Handbook No. 8-1, by Consumer and Food Economics Institute (Washington, D.C.: Agricultural Research Service, U.S. Department of Agriculture, 1976).

Page 33

"Calories at the Cocktail Hour" adapted from *Bowes and Church's Food Values of Portions Commonly Used*, 13th ed., by Jean A. T. Pennington and Helen Nichols Church (New York: Harper & Row, 1980)
and
Nutritive Value of American Foods in Common Units, Agriculture Handbook No. 456, by Catherine F. Adams (Washington, D.C.: Agricultural Research Service, U.S. Department of Agriculture, 1975)
and
Provisional Table on the Nutrient Content of Canned Vegetables and Vegetable Products, by Consumer and Food Economics Institute (Hyattsville, Md.: Science and Education Administration, U.S. Department of Agriculture, 1979)
and
Composition of Foods: Fruit and Fruit Juices, Agriculture Handbook No. 8-9, by Consumer Nutrition Center (Washington, D.C.: Human Nutrition Information Service, U.S. Department of Agriculture, 1982).

Chapter 5

Page 82

"Don't Let Sugar Sneak Up on You" adapted from "Too Much Sugar?", *Consumer Reports*, March, 1978.

Chapter 7

Page 108

"Charting Your Progress" adapted from *Maximum Personal Energy*, by Charles T. Kuntzleman (Emmaus, Pa.: Rodale Press, 1981).

Chapter 9

Page 142

"Why Fasting Fails" adapted from *Nutrition, Weight Control, and Exercise*, 2d ed., by Frank I. Katch and William D. McArdle (Philadelphia: Lea & Febiger, 1983)
and
"Nutrition and Energy Balance in Body Composition Studies," by Francisco Grande, in *Techniques for Measuring Body Composition*, Josef Brozek and Austin Henschel, eds. (Washington, D.C.: National Academy of Sciences—National Research Council, 1961). Reprinted by permission of the publisher.

Page 150

"Maintaining Your Loss" adapted from *The Partnership Diet Program* by Kelly D. Brownell with Irene Copeland (New York: Rawson, Wade Publishers, 1980). Reprinted by permission of the publisher and author.

Chapter 10

Pages 154-163

"Your Calorie Counter" adapted from *Nutritive Value of American Foods in Common Units*, Agriculture Handbook No. 456, by Catherine F. Adams (Washington, D.C.: Agricultural Research Service, U.S. Department of Agriculture, 1975)
and
Composition of Foods: Fruits and Fruit Juices, Agriculture Handbook No. 8-9, by Consumer Nutrition Center (Washington, D.C.: Human Nutrition Information Service, U.S. Department of Agriculture, 1982)
and
Composition of Foods: Breakfast Cereals, Agriculture Handbook No. 8-8, by Consumer Nutrition Center (Washington, D.C.: Human Nutrition Information Service, U.S. Department of Agriculture, 1982)
and
Composition of Foods: Soups, Sauces and Gravies, Agriculture Handbook No. 8-6, by Consumer and Food Economics Institute (Washington, D.C.: Science and Education Administration, U.S. Department of Agriculture, 1980)
and
Composition of Foods: Dairy and Egg Products, Agriculture Handbook No. 8-1, by Consumer and Food Economics Institute (Washington, D.C.: Agricultural Research Service, U.S. Department of Agriculture, 1976)
and
Composition of Foods: Sausages and Luncheon Meats, Agriculture Handbook No. 8-7, by Consumer Nutrition Center (Washington, D.C.: Science and Education Administration, U.S. Department of Agriculture, 1980)
and
Composition of Foods: Poultry Products, Agriculture Handbook No. 8-5, by Consumer and Food Economics Institute (Washington, D.C.: Science and Education Administration, U.S. Department of Agriculture, 1979)
and
Proximate Composition of Beef from Carcass to Cooked Meat: Method of Derivation and Tables of Values, Home Economics Research Report No. 31, by Consumer and Food Economics Division (Washington, D.C.: Agricultural Research Service, U.S. Depart-

ment of Agriculture, 1972)
and
Bowes and Church's Food Values of Portions Commonly Used, 13th ed., by Jean A. T. Pennington and Helen Nichols Church (New York: Harper & Row, 1980)
and
Provisional Table on the Nutrient Content of Canned Vegetables and Vegetable Products, by Consumer and Food Economics Institute (Hyattsville, Md.: Science and Education Administration, U.S. Department of Agriculture, 1979)
and
Provisional Table on the Nutrient Content of Beverages, by Nutrient Data Research Group, Consumer Nutrition Center (Washington, D.C.: Human Nutrition Information Service, U.S. Department of Agriculture, 1982)
and
Composition of Foods: Pork Products, Agriculture Handbook No. 8-10, by Consumer Nutrition Division (Washington, D.C.: Human Nutrition Information Service, U.S. Deparmtent of Agriculture, 1983)
and
Provisional Table on the Nutrient Content of Frozen Vegetables, by Consumer and Food Economics Institute (Hyattsville, Md.: Science and Education Administration, U.S. Department of Agriculture, 1979)
and
Nutritive Value of Foods, Home and Garden Bulletin No. 72, by Consumer and Food Economics Institute (Washington, D.C.: Science and Education Administration, U.S. Department of Agriculture, 1978)
and
Composition of Foods: Fats and Oils, Agriculture Handbook No. 8-4, by Consumer and Food Economics Institute (Washington, D.C.:

Science and Education Administration, U.S. Department of Agriculture, 1979)
and
"Nutrient Content of Canned Legumes," by G. A. Halaby, R. W. Lewis and C. R. Rey, *Food Technology*, March, 1981
and
"The Glycaemic Index of Foods Tested in Diabetic Patients: A New Basis for Carbohydrate Exchange Favouring the Use of Legumes," by D. J. A. Jenkins et al, *Diabetologia*, April, 1983.

Photography Credits

Cover: Margaret Skrovanek
Staff Photographers—
Christopher Barone: pp. viii-1; 10, top; 11, bottom; 26; 27; 31; 32-33; 60-61; 86-87; 190, top left. Angelo M. Caggiano: pp. 40, bottom; 41; 54, bottom; 55; 74-75; 104-105. Carl Doney: pp. 42, bottom; 43; 44; 45; 46, bottom; 47; 50, bottom; 51; 81; 109, top right; 109, bottom center; 122-123; 148. T. L. Gettings: pp. 108, center and bottom. Mitchell T. Mandel: pp 21; 42, top; 56, right; 57; 58, bottom; 59; 63; 153. Alison Miksch: pp. 22; 94-95. Scott Schmidt: pp. 104-105. Margaret Skrovanek: pp.10, bottom; 16-17; 39; 80; 96; 102-103; 108, top; 109, top center; 116-117; 132-133; 149. Christie C. Tito: pp. 84-85; 111; 138-139. Sally Shenk Ullman: pp. 24-25; 28-29; 36-37; 48, bottom; 49; 52, bottom; 53; 69; 71; 110; 119; 129; 154-155. Rodale Press Photography Dept.: p. 99.

Other Photographers—
Willy Bogner/The Image Bank: p. 107. Casarena/FPG International: pp. 76-77. Jeff Cox: p. 40, top. Cynthia Foster/First Foto Bank: p. 56, left. Donna Kruetz: pp. 116, top left; 117, top right; 118; 120. David Lissy/FPG International: p. 5, bottom left. J. Messerschmidt/Bruce Coleman,

Inc.: p. 46, top. Robert Rodale: p. 50, top. Pat Seip: p. 109, bottom. Raeanne Rubenstein/PEOPLE Weekly (copyright 1982 Time, Inc.): p. 91. S. Vidler/Leo de Wys, Inc.: pp. 48, top; 52, top; 54, top. Jonathan Wright/Bruce Coleman, Inc.: p. 58, top.

Additional Photographs Courtesy of—The Bettman Archive, Inc.: pp. 4, right; 5, right. Culver Pictures: pp. 4, top right and center; 5, top left. GAF Corporation: p. 3. The Guinness Book of World Records (copyright 1983 Sterling Publishing Co., Inc.): p. 11. Photo World/FPG International: p. 9.

Food Styling Credits

Barbara Fritz: pp. 28-29; 32-33; 36-37; 40, bottom; 41; 48, bottom; 49. Kay Seng Lichthardt: pp. viii-1; 32-33; 46, bottom; 47; 50, bottom; 51, 52, bottom; 53; 54, bottom; 55; 63; 71; 119; 122-123; 154-155. Laura Hendry Reifsnyder: pp. 31; 42, bottom; 43; 44; 45; 58, bottom; 59; 69. Kathryn Sommons: pp. 86-87. Elinor Wilson: pp. 56, right; 57.

Recipes developed by—
Anita Hirsch, JoAnn Coponi, Rhonda Diehl, Linda Gilbert, of the Rodale Test Kitchen, and Nancy J. Ayers, Susan Burwell, Lynn Cohen, Debra Deis, Marie Harrington, Ann Sheridan, Michael Stoner.

Illustration Credits

Bascove: pp. 126; 127; 156; 157; 158; 159; 160; 161; 162; 163. Susan M. Blubaugh: pp. 97; 130; 141. Joe Lertola: pp. 2; 8; 13; 23; 66-67; 72; 88; 92; 150-151. Donna Ruff: pp. 18; 64; 65; 136; 140. Mary Anne Shea: pp. 6; 12; 78-79; 93; 112-113; 124; 125; 134.

Special Thanks to—
"Breezy," Fleetwood, Pa.; Brocato and Kelman, Inc., Los Angeles; Brookstone's, Peterborough, N.H.; Creative

Resources, New York; Life Power Products, Los Angeles; Schoen's Furniture, Allentown, Pa.: Spymark, Vista, Calif.; Ye Olde Tuxedo Shoppe, Emmaus, Pa.

Index

Rodale Press, Inc., publishes PREVENTION®, the better health magazine.
For information on how to order your subscription,
write to PREVENTION®, Emmaus, PA 18049.